# METHODOLOGICAL APPROACHES TO THE STUDY OF BRAIN MATURATION AND ITS ABNORMALITIES

**Summary Report**
of a symposium held May 11- 12, 1971, co-sponsored by the Rose F. Kennedy Center
for Research in Mental Retardation and Human Development, Albert Einstein College of Medicine, Yeshiva University; and the Mental Retardation Program of the
National Institute of Child Health and Human Development, National Institutes of
Health, United States Public Health Service.

*NICHD — Mental Retardation Research Centers Series*

# Methodological Approaches to the Study of Brain Maturation and its Abnormalities

Scientific Editors:
**Dominick P. Purpura, M.D.**
Director
Rose F. Kennedy Center for Research in
Mental Retardation and Human Development

and
**Georgia Perkins Reaser, M.D.**
Special Assistant to the Director
National Institute of Child Health
and Human Development

Technical Editor:
**Anne H. Rosenfeld**

UNIVERSITY PARK PRESS

Baltimore • London • Tokyo

UNIVERSITY PARK PRESS
International Publishers in Science and Medicine
Chamber of Commerce Building
Baltimore, Maryland 21202

*616.8*

*m 56*

*66088*

**Library of Congress Cataloging in Publication Data**
Main entry under title:

Methodological approaches to the study of brain maturation
and its abnormalities.

"A symposium held May 11-12, 1971, co-sponsored by the Rose F. Kennedy Center for Research in Mental Retardation and Human Development, Albert Einstein College of Medicine, Yeshiva University; and the Mental Retardation Program of the National Institute of Child Health and Human Development, National Institutes of Health, PHS."

Bibliography: p.

1. Brain—Anatomy—Congresses. 2. Developmental psychobiology—Congresses. 3. Brain—Abnormities and deformities—Congresses. 4. Neurology— Technique—Congresses. I. Purpura, Dominick P., ed. II. Rose F. Kennedy Center for Research in Mental Retardation and Human Development. III. United States. National Institute of Child Health and Human Development. Mental Retardation Branch. [DNLM: 1. Brain—Abnormalities—Congresses. 2. Brain—Growth & development—Congresses. 3. Mental retardation—Etiology—Congresses. WM300 M592 1971]
RJ492.M47          616.8'588'071          73-10081
ISBN 0-8391-0717-X

# Contents

# Participants

**M. V. L. Bennett, D. Phil.**
Department of Anatomy
Albert Einstein College of Medicine
Rose F. Kennedy Center for Re-
search in Mental Retardation and
Human Development
1410 Pelham Parkway South
Bronx, New York 10461

**Sidney W. Bijou, Ph.D.**
Department of Psychology
University of Illinois
403 East Healy
Champaign, Illinois 61820

**Herbert G. Birch, M.D., Ph.D.***
Department of Pediatrics
Albert Einstein College of Medicine
Rose F. Kennedy Center for Re-
search in Mental Retardation and
Human Development
1410 Pelham Parkway South
Bronx, New York 10461

**Murray B. Bornstein, M.D.**
Department of Neurology
Albert Einstein College of Medicine
Rose F. Kennedy Center for Re-
search in Mental Retardation and
Human Development
1410 Pelham Parkway South
Bronx, New York 10461

**B. G. Cragg, Ph.D.**
Department of Physiology
Monash University
Clayton, Victoria, Australia

**Stanley M. Crain, Ph.D.**
Department of Physiology
Albert Einstein College of Medicine
Rose F. Kennedy Center for Re-
search in Mental Retardation and
Human Development
1410 Pelham Parkway South
Bronx, New York 10461

**Sibylle Escalona, Ph.D.**
Department of Psychiatry
Albert Einstein College of Medicine
Rose F. Kennedy Center for Re-
search in Mental Retardation and
Human Development
1410 Pelham Parkway South
Bronx, New York 10461

**Harry H. Gordon, M.D.**
Department of Pediatrics
Albert Einstein College of Medicine
Director Emeritus, Rose F. Kennedy
Center for Research in Mental
Retardation and Human Devel-
opment
1410 Pelham Parkway South
Bronx, New York 10461

*Deceased.

**Gerard M. Lehrer, M.D.**
Department of Neurology
Mount Sinai School of Medicine
Fifth Avenue & 100th Street
New York, New York 10029

**Lewis P. Lipsitt, Ph.D.**
Department of Psychology
Brown University
Providence, Rhode Island 02912

**Guy McKhann, M.D.**
Department of Neurology
Johns Hopkins University
School of Medicine
725 N. Wolfe Street
Baltimore, Maryland 21205

**Gilbert W. Meier, Ph.D.**
Department of Psychology
John F. Kennedy Center for
Research
George Peabody College for
Teachers
Nashville, Tennessee 97203

**William T. Norton, Ph.D.**
Department of Neurology
Albert Einstein College of Medicine
1300 Morris Park Avenue
Bronx, New York 10461

**George D. Pappas, Ph.D.**
Department of Anatomy
Albert Einstein College of Medicine
1300 Morris Park Avenue
Bronx, New York 10461

**Dominick P. Purpura, M.D.**
Professor and Chairman of the Department of Anatomy
Albert Einstein College of Medicine
Director, Rose F. Kennedy Center
for Research in Mental Retardation and Human Development
1410 Pelham Parkway South
Bronx, New York 10461

**Norman S. Radin, Ph.D.**
Mental Health Research Institute
University of Michigan
205 N. Forest Avenue
Ann Arbor, Michigan 48104

**Michael Shelanski, M.D.**
Laboratory of Biochemical Genetics
National Heart Institute
National Institutes of Health
Bethesda, Maryland 20014

**Eric M. Shooter, Ph.D., D.Sc.**
Department of Genetics
Stanford University Medical School
Stanford, California 94305

**Gerald Turkewitz, Ph.D.**
Department of Pediatrics
Albert Einstein College of Medicine
Rose F. Kennedy Center for Re-
search in Mental Retardation and
Human Development
1410 Pelham Parkway South
Bronx, New York 10461

**Hendrik Van der Loos, M.D.**
Department of Anatomy
Johns Hopkins University
School of Medicine
725 N. Wolfe Street
Baltimore, Maryland 21205

**Herbert Vaughan, M.D.**
Department of Neurology
Albert Einstein College of Medicine
Rose F. Kennedy Center for Research in Mental Retardation and Human Development
1410 Pelham Parkway South
Bronx, New York 10461

**Myron Winick, M.D.**
Department of Pediatrics
The New York Hospital
525 East 68th Street
New York, New York 10021

**M. Kenneth Wolf, M.D.**
Department of Anatomy
University of Massachusetts Medical School
55 Lake Avenue North
Worcester, Massachusetts 01605

# Preface

This report summarizes the results of a two-day symposium (May 11-12, 1971) co-sponsored by the Mental Retardation Program of the National Institute of Child Health and Human Development and the Rose F. Kennedy Center for Research in Mental Retardation and Human Development, Albert Einstein College of Medicine, Yeshiva University. This symposium was the third in a continuing series of Mental Retardation Research Center conferences. The first, at the University of Kansas Center, was concerned with the language of the retarded; the second, at the University of Chicago, dealt with antenatal diagnosis. Through these Mental Retardation Research Center conferences, the Institute hopes to facilitate scientific communication among all scientists, whether working within the centers or on the national or international scene. Through such lines of communication, new scientific data emerging from laboratories and clinics throughout the world should become readily accessible to all workers concerned with basic research into the causes of mental retardation. Hopefully, this will facilitate a more concerted attack on the problems of diagnosis and clinical management of the mentally retarded.

Gerald D. LaVeck, M.D.
Director
National Institute of Child Health
and Human Development

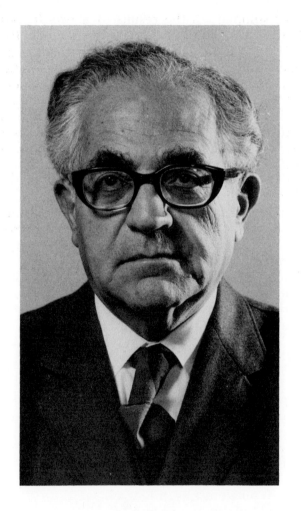

Harry H. Gordon, M.D.

# Foreword

It is fitting that research methodology for studying the maturation of the brain and behavior should be the subject of one of the first interdisciplinary conferences to be held at the Rose F. Kennedy Center for Research in Mental Retardation and Human Development. Neurological deficits in prematurely born infants, mental retardation, and other developmental disabilities and aberrant behavioral development are all serious clinical problems in infants and children. They color not only the children's lives, but those of their siblings and parents as well. They cry out for solution because of the physical and emotional suffering and the financial costs that they incur.

New basic knowledge and methods of application are needed to prevent the occurrence or to mitigate the severity of developmental disabilities. In the final analysis, there must be more basic knowledge of the developing nervous system. The nervous system is the common substrate in which a variety of insults wreak their havoc, whether they are inborn errors of metabolism or prenatal or postnatal insults from the environment, such as viral diseases, poverty, emotional deprivation, lead poisoning, battering by parents, or automobile accidents.

The report of the President's Panel on Mental Retardation was converted into Public Law 88-164 and signed by President Kennedy in October, 1963. This law provided funds for construction of centers for research in mental retardation and related aspects of human development; for construction of university-affiliated centers, the primary responsibility of which would be training of personnel in new methods of care of the retarded; and for community services to the retarded. The efforts on behalf of the retarded are much greater now than they were before the report of the President's Panel. Since then, there have been gradual implementation of the construction program and continuing support of research, service, and training programs even though the needs are still great for large segments of the retarded population.

Thanks are due to the continuing efforts of the staffs of the National Institute of Child Health and Human Development, other constituents of the National Institutes of Health, the Health Service and Mental Health Administration, additional Divisions of the Public Health Service, the Children's Bureau, and the Office of Education, the President's Committee on Mental Retardation, and associations of parents, such as the National Association for Retarded Children and its various state components. These associations continue to fight so that retarded children shall not be the "least of these," but shall have human rights as human beings.

The Rose F. Kennedy Center is proud to be able to participate in a great national effort which is in the better, not worse, traditions of our country. It is an integral part of the Albert Einstein College of Medicine of Yeshiva University. It is physically and functionally connected to the Jacobi Hospital, the main hospital of the Bronx Municipal Hospital Center, particularly in the high-risk newborn infants' and obstetric services as well as the out-patient clinics. The major emphases of the scientific activities inside the Kennedy Center are research and research training; the major emphases of the clinic and outreach programs are service and service training. The research programs are multidisciplinary, in a milieu designed to permit the development of interdisciplinary programs on an operational rather than administrative basis. For example, a pediatrician who is studying the effect of phototherapy on hyperbilirubinemia has the cooperation of a clinical scientist with a background in clinical neurophysiology and behavior who is using the electroencephalogram to study the effects of phototherapy.

The laboratory research programs give major emphasis to developmental neurobiology, including neurophysiology, ultrastructure, and biochemistry; neuropathology; biochemical and cytological genetics; behavioral sciences; developmental physiology, including respiratory, renal, hepatic, and endocrine sections; and human ecology. The clinical facilities of the center consist of a clinical research unit for both prolonged observations on in-patients and short-term observations on ambulatory patients. Children with neurological problems such as mental retardation, persistent seizures, or communication disorders have been admitted, as well as children with inborn errors of metabolism and endocrine or neuroendocrine problems. Normal and high-risk newborn infants have been transferred to the Center for sleep studies. Short-term observations such as insulin and growth hormone assays, as well as renal clearances, have been made in children with developmental disabilities. The Clinical Research Unit is expected to be of major importance in evaluating various types of intervention in children with developmental disabilities who are referred by the Children's Evaluation and Rehabilitation Clinic, one of our other main clinical resources.

The Children's Evaluation and Rehabilitation Clinic is the major diagnostic and evaluation center for the Bronx, a borough with 1.5 million population. This center is critical in clinical research programs, such as careful long-term follow-up studies of premature infants with different levels of tyrosinemia; a study of the relation of dental enamel injury to time of insult; a study of home management of motor handicaps such as those of cerebral palsy; a study of reading disabilities in a neighboring public school; and a study in collaboration with our Social Ecology Research Unit on the delivery of service in the Genetic Counselling Clinic and the Children's Evaluation and Rehabilitation Clinic. The Social Ecology Unit also has counselled the architects for the new Bronx State School and, with the new director, who is a member of our Kennedy staff, plans to set up methods for the evaluation of community services for the retarded.

The Children's Evaluation and Rehabilitation Clinic also has served as a facility for training pediatric and dental house officers, nurses, psychologists, and social workers in the special problems of retarded children.

Our Center is thus a combination of a mental retardation research center and a university diagnostic and evaluation center which provides training and articulates with the community. The broad range of activities in research thus encompasses studies of cells, organs, animals, and retarded children and their families and communities. As the first Center under

Public Law 88-164, we try to fulfill the law's promise and that of Congress to the taxpayers on behalf of some of the most needy: the mentally retarded. In supplying new knowledge and personnel, we also try to be worthy of the great lady whose name graces our building.

Harry H. Gordon, M.D.
Director Emeritus
Rose F. Kennedy Center

NARC-Grover F. Powers
Professor of Pediatrics
Albert Einstein College of
Medicine, Yeshiva University

# Overview

In the earliest phases of embryonic development, differentiation of ectodermal elements occurs to form the neural crest. Some 30 years later the morphological maturation of the brain is completed when intrahemispheric association pathways acquire their full complement of myelin. Throughout this prolonged period of brain maturation, but notably in late fetal stages and the first few years, the immature brain is particularly vulnerable to disturbances which may be impressed by genetic abnormalities, trauma, or other perturbations of the external or internal environment. How these various factors contribute to deficiencies in information processing, disorders of sensorimotor integration and language capability, and other disturbances of "higher nervous activities" remains unclarified. What is clear, however, is that further definition of this problem is essential if an adequate understanding of the nature of mental subnormality (in the broadest sense of the term) is to be attained. That there can be no single all-embracing methodological approach to this problem is self-evident. This follows from the painful fact that there is no common currency for information exchange across the borders of semiautonomous or sovereign scientific disciplines.

The neuromorphologist deals with the structure of membranes, subcellular organelles, synapses, neurons, and neuronal subsystems of varying complexity. The neurophysiologist is concerned largely with electrical signs of neuronal function and integration and perhaps with attempts to relate electrophysiological activities of single neurons or variable populations of neurons to distinct but partial elements of simple behaviors. The neurochemist deals with the metabolic machinery and chemical nature of the structural components of neurons and glia. However romantic the notion of macromolecular control of modifications of neuronal functions may be, the link between molecular biology and nervous system functions remains tenuous at best. For the most part, the investigator interested in behaving organisms deals with global concepts such as learning, cognition, motivation, and reward usually without reference to discrete morphophysiological and biochemical phenomena. A possible exception to this may be those studies in which complex behavioral activities may be triggered or released by pharmacological activation (or inhibition) of discrete neuronal subsystems. Even in these studies, major questions of the nature and site of drug actions and specificity of responsiveness have been addressed only tentatively.

The language of each discipline constituting the "brain and behavioral sciences" has its own deep structure, and much of what is meaningful in one discipline may be lost in translation to another. There is as much a need to overcome language barriers between even closely related disciplines as there is to explore new depths of knowledge in a particular narrowly focused area of investigation. Yet the hot pursuit of well-defined problems in a particular discipline (or subdiscipline) has yielded the most general principles of biology. Such an approach is not likely to be forsaken by any save the most foolhardy, or the most courageous, depending upon one's point of view.

What scientists do well, for the most part, is to identify a problem, pose a question, develop a technology for making controlled observations, and then, if data are generated, pose suitable hypotheses for further exploration of the problem. Not infrequently, however, advances in understanding of particular problems follow upon the heels of major technological developments. Clearly, the electron microscope was not invented to study the fine structure of the nervous system. However, the availability of this instrument has revolutionized and galvanized research in neurobiology. Unfortunately, not all technological advances have had such salutary effects. Computers of various sizes and complexity are by now essential tools for neurophysiological and behavioral studies. However, the disappointing results obtained to date in attempts to apply computerized profile-recognition techniques to the analysis of neuronal connectivity patterns in the mammalian brain amply attest to the sterility of research programs generated largely by the availability of machines in search of a function. Fortunately, this trend may be reversed as more clearly defined studies of connectivity patterns in simple invertebrate neuronal systems become amenable to computer analysis.

Technology is but one facet of a methodological approach in science. Other facets reflect research strategies that include considerations of effort, availability of materials, feasibility of success, and preparation for uncertainty. Of these, only the last requires very special training in the art of adjusting to disappointments. Few practice this well; hence the avoidance principle: avoid that which is not part of one's practical universe of discourse. After all, morphology is the proper domain of the well-trained morphologist and the same applies in kind to the physiologist, biochemist, etc. Doing one's own thing, *well*, has never been considered counter-productive. Indeed, such behavior on the part of the energetic bench scientist has been handsomely rewarded traditionally and should continue to receive the highest priority by funding agencies. Perhaps the expectation here is that every so often genetic recombination in the training of specialists in a particular discipline will yield a "Renaissance man" capable of productive scientific enterprise in a number of disciplines. The ever-present danger, however, is that marriages between disciplines may result in cross-disciplinary sterilization!

The problem of specifying and evaluating the methodological approaches that are likely to contribute to an understanding of the morphophysiological, biochemical, and psychological bases of mental subnormality addresses all the foregoing issues. Each discipline of the brain and behavioral sciences has its own history, tradition, language, special techniques, and subcultural fetishes. Apropos of the latter, the preparation of "good" microelectrodes for intracellular recording from neurons constitutes a highly personal endeavor compounded of luck and skill in varying proportions. Yet so much of the ultimate value of this approach to the study of neuronal organization depends upon the availability of "good" microelectrodes that progress in this area of neurobiological investigation may be dependent upon the rate-limiting step of making suitable micropipettes! Anyone who has attempted to utilize the various Golgi methods for studying the development of neurons encounters the same hidden obstructions to progress. Nothing in the neurobiological sciences requires more patience and prayer than the preparation of "good" Golgi material. No amount of close adherence to textbook description of "How to Make Golgi Preparations" (or "How to Make Ultramicropipettes") can take the place of experience, patience, and supplication to appropriate gods. Unfortunately, there is a tendency to avoid discussions of methodological difficulties in the description of new experimental data. Obviously, such information is as valuable as the nature of the data themselves. This brings us to the aims and objectives of the symposium on "Methodological Approaches to the Study of Brain Maturation and Its Abnormalities," which is summarized in the following pages.

The genesis of this symposium may be traced from consideration of the several issues noted above, which include the need to define precisely the nature of available methods, their advantages and limitations, and the manner by which such methods may be applied to the central problem of studies of brain maturation and its abnormalities. In addition, it was hoped that a common purpose served by different methodologies could set the stage for developing more coherent multidisciplinary research efforts. It was recognized from the outset that unless precautions were taken to limit the presentation of *new* data, probably none of these issues would be sufficiently explored in depth. Thus the charge to the participants in preparing their discussions explicitly precluded extensive data presentation. Stripped of the usual supporting props of data-bearing slides, each participant was then asked to recount the rationale for his or her particular methodological approach and to define its limits of usefulness. In some instances, discussants seized the opportunity to criticize available methodologies and to suggest priorities for the development of new methods and technological equipment. The search for new models and their applicability to studies of normal brain maturation and of clinical disorders was also highlighted by several participants. Suffice it to say that some found it impossible to adhere to the charge of the organizing committee. Their presentations were the usual data-packed, rapid-fire displays which related to specific research topics. What was patently obvious from this is how intellectually stimulating it is to plunge across new research frontiers—and how difficult it is to examine, reflect upon, and criticize the means to the end and the nature of the objective itself.

The casual reader of this Summary Report who seeks to discover new insights into the normal and pathological processes of brain maturation will find little here to satisfy this curiosity. On the other hand, the experienced laboratory and clinical investigator knows too well the various problems raised in discussion of different methodologies to benefit greatly from another cataloging of these approaches. Hopefully, however, a redefinition of purposes, methods, and procedures may serve to catalyze a host of reactions, not the least of which may be the recognition that stimulus-bound behavior prejudices us in favor of our own precious methodological approaches.

Dominick P. Purpura, M.D.
Director
Rose F. Kennedy Center for
Research in Mental Retardation
and Human Development

# SESSION I.
# STUDIES OF SIMPLE NEURONAL SYSTEMS

# Tissue Culture Techniques: General Remarks

**M. Bornstein**

Although the first subject area examined in the symposium was concerned with simple neuronal systems, the session chairman, Dr. M. Bornstein, recognized at the outset that probably no experimental model could be justifiably considered to meet this requirement. Nevertheless, he noted that many investigators have utilized tissue culture of the nervous system as an effective, relatively simplified approach to salient problems of developmental neurobiology.

Dr. Bornstein traced the origins of the tissue culture approach as applied to the nervous system to the beginning of this century when Harrison first explanted a fragment of frog spinal cord and noted the outgrowth of neurites. His work gave considerable support to the unitary theory of the neuron. Characterization of the various cells that migrated from fragments of nerve tissue maintained in culture proceeded in the 1930's and 1940's notably in the laboratories of Pomerat and Hogue. Much of the present day perfection of the Maximow slide technique and its application to nervous tissue may be traced to the work of Murray and her associates, particularly in studies with Peterson.

The Maximow slide is simply a glass depression slide over which a square cover slip is sealed. A round cover slip is enclosed which carries the cultured fragment, usually obtained from an embryo or newborn animal. The advantage of the Maximow slide technique is that it permits periodic observations of the tissue during its entire *in vitro* existence. Cultures prepared in this fashion may be examined for months and occasionally for years. Observations can be made on the differentiation and maturation of various components of the tissue while at the same time permitting the investigator to manipulate the environment of the tissue.

The nervous system differs in several major respects from other organ systems, particularly in the establishment of relationships between elements at macroscopic and microscopic levels. Two of the most obvious intercellular relationships are evident in myelin formation between glia and neurons and in synapse formation between neuron and neuron or neuron and muscle (smooth and striated).

In the early 1950's, Peterson (then in Murray's laboratory) first demonstrated myelin formation in cultured chick embryo dorsal root ganglia. Peterson's techniques are now widely employed in many laboratories in studies of peripheral nervous tissue. In recent investigations carried out at the Albert Einstein College of Medicine, Peterson has explanted fragments of spinal cord and skeletal muscle separately and has noted the sequential events during the formation of neuromuscular junctions. Of particular interest is the observation that such junctions may be formed between spinal cord and muscle fragments from different species. Thus rodent spinal cord has been coupled to fragments of human adult muscle obtained at biopsy. According to Dr. Bornstein, since important trophic influences can be shown to develop between the nerve and muscle, this technique offers a considerable advantage in pursuing problems of trophic relationships at synapses.

The Maximow slide technique has also been applied to central nervous system (CNS) tissues. Hild was the first to demonstrate myelin formation in mammalian CNS in cultures of newborn kitten cerebellum maintained in a roller tube on a flying cover slip. The cover slip can be removed from the roller tube and the tissues examined at high magnification. Unfortunately, the roller tube method does not allow the prolonged, continuous observation of tissues throughout their entire *in vitro* existence which is permitted by the Maximow slide technique.

Myelin is produced in culture by neuroglial cells, primarily oligodendroglia. Electron microscopy of cultured tissues indicates that myelin is formed by neuroglial cell membrane fusions, as is the case *in vivo*. The problem of myelinogenesis can be attacked along several lines. For example, myelin formation can be inhibited in the presence of antiserum directed against the central nervous system. Both the differentiation of glial cells to oligodendrocytes and the formation of myelin can be inhibited indefinitely in the presence of antiserum. When the antiserum is removed from the culture, however, glial differentiation and myelin formation resume within a few days. Such studies permit an opportunity to undertake biochemical studies of the inhibited and disinhibited tissues, as summarized in Dr. Lehrer's presentation *(vide infra)*.

A number of advances have taken place in recent years in the tissue culture of virtually all neuraxial sites, including the cerebral neocortex. This has led to a new line of inquiry concerning the *in vitro* development of synaptic relations between fragments of nervous tissue taken from different neuraxial locations. Functional and morphological synaptic relations have now been demonstrated between fragments of spinal cord and brain stem and between brain stem and cerebral neocortex.

Dr. Bornstein cited one study carried out with his associates which is particularly relevant to the question of the relationship between function and morphological features of developing synaptic systems. In this study an attempt was made to influence the development of synapses in cultured CNS tissue by maintaining the tissue from the time of explantation (when no synapses were evident electrophysiologically or ultrastructurally) in an environment which would abolish bioelectrical activity and impulse propagation as recorded by extracellularly located electrodes. Additional details of the methods employed are summarized elsewhere in this report. Suffice it to say that in the presence of pharmacological agents capable of suppressing bioelectrical activity in the cultures, synapse formation proceeded unimpeded. Upon removal of the suppressing agents (xylocaine and magnesium), marked and immediate polysynaptic responses were elicited in studies by Dr. Crain.

In summarizing the general usefulness of the tissue culture method, Dr. Bornstein emphasized the wide variety of alterations that could be produced in the environment of cultured fragments. Such manipulations might include addition of metabolites, antimetabolites, viruses, antibodies, and bacterial toxins. The possibility of developing suitable techniques for examining problems of neuronal recognition, and transmitter, neurohumoral, and neuroendocrine phenomena in tissue culture amply attests to the power of the technique.

# Tissue Culture Models of Maturing Brain Functions

S. M. Crain

The availability of a variety of cultured subsystems of CNS tissues has made it feasible to apply neurophysiological, neuropharmacological, and neuromorphological techniques to the continuing *in vitro* study of the developing nervous system.

During the past two decades, Dr. Crain and his associates have been carrying out a variety of physiological studies of neural cultures to gain insights into mechanisms of growth and function of neurons that may be difficult to study in the living animal. This technique greatly facilitates direct experimental control and manipulation of the physicochemical environment of nerve cells. Since *embryonic* neural tissues adapt best to culture conditions, these *in vitro* preparations are useful model systems for various problems in developmental neurobiology, e.g., electrogenesis, development of axonal conductile properties, and synaptogenesis.

A number of laboratories have recently begun to focus on electrogenesis in connection with neuroblastoma cultures. Nelson et al. (1969, 1971), for example, have shown that under certain conditions *in vitro* primitive neuroblastoma cells may sprout axons which can generate characteristic action potentials. Since large quantities of membrane can be obtained from these rapidly growing cells, the material may lend itself to characterization of critical chemical factors associated with the development of conductile membranes in these clones. Similar phenomena occur during the early outgrowth of nerve fibers after explantation of normal embryonic neural tissues, e.g., dorsal root ganglia, spinal cord, or cerebral cortex. The axons severed during surgical isolation of the neural tissue regenerate *in vitro*, and many of the shorter intact neurons in the explant continue to grow arborizing neurites as in normal embryonic development. The earliest stages of onset of conductile activity can, therefore, be studied in the newly grown or regenerated axons of these primary neural cultures, but the quantity of membranes available for correlative biochemical analyses is, of course, far less than in neuroblastoma cultures.

The great advantage of the primary neural tissue cultures is the remarkable degree of *intercellular* organization which can develop after explantation of immature CNS tissues. Not only does conductile activity appear within the individual axons during the first few days *in vitro,* but as these axons arborize they form characteristic synaptic junctions with one another leading to generation of complex bioelectric activities (Crain, 1966, 1970a; Crain and Peterson, 1967). Dr. Crain described some of the bioelectrical activities of these cultures which indicate not only the occurrence of synaptogenesis in many explanted neurons, but also evidence of the formation of ordered, patterned synaptic networks. Complex, yet stereotyped, discharge patterns develop during maturation of these CNS tissues *in vitro* resembling types of CNS activities *in situ* which appear to be due to sequential activation of excitatory and inhibitory synaptic components in highly ordered neuronal networks. These complex synaptic discharge patterns can be triggered by local electrical stimuli applied to the cultured tissue; many of the CNS explants also show interesting rhythms, with cycles ranging from tenths of seconds to several minutes. Some of these complex spontaneous rhythmical discharges resemble embryonic motility patterns. These types of CNS cultures may be useful for studies of mechanisms underlying the onset and development of primitive behavior (Corner and Crain, 1969, 1972, Crain, 1973a).

Organotypic cultures are obviously quite complex systems and, as Dr. Crain pointed out, it may be somewhat misleading to include them in a discussion of "simple neuronal systems." They are, however, simple in the sense that they are composed of only a small fraction of the cells generally involved in comparable functional studies *in situ.* CNS explants are, in fact, only about 1 mm$^3$ in size, probably containing a few hundred neurons embedded in a complex neuroglial meshwork. They are also simple in the sense that the excitable neural tissues are relatively unsheathed and accessible to experimental manipulation of the environment. Problems analogous to the "blood-brain barrier" are far less serious in these explants, and large macromolecules which normally would not be expected to get through to CNS neurons *in situ* can be made readily accessible to the cultured nerve cells. Antibodies, for example, have now been fruitfully used as selective immunopharmacological agents to block bioelectrical activities in CNS cultures studied as model systems in relation to multiple sclerosis (Bornstein and Crain, 1965, 1971; Carnegie, 1971).

Cerebral neocortex tissues explanted from fetal or neonatal mice have provided a particularly interesting model for developmental studies (Crain, 1964; Crain and Bornstein, 1964). During the first few days *in vitro* only simple brief spike potentials can be evoked by electrical stimuli applied to the cerebral explants (Fig. 1*A*). The neurons can evidently generate and propagate action potentials but no signs of complex responses indicative of synaptic network activity have been detected at this early stage. By 4 days *in vitro*, however, similar local stimuli may trigger long-lasting barrages of spikes as well as complex patterned slow wave responses with long latencies (Fig. 1*B*). The latter potentials become larger in amplitude and somewhat shorter in duration during the ensuing week of maturation *in vitro* (Figs. 1*C* and 2$A_{2-4}$), and they can be greatly enhanced with strychnine. Microelectrode recordings of the long-lasting potentials evoked from superficial (pial) regions of these cerebral cortical explants (Fig. 1, *lower section*) often show characteristic negative polarity (Figs. 1*B*, 1*C*, and 2$A_{2-4}$: *upper sweeps*), whereas potentials recorded simultaneously from "deep" loci tend to be positive and even longer in latency and duration (Figs. 1*B*, 1*C*, and 2$A_{2-4}$: *lower sweeps*). The temporal patterns and polarity properties of these extracellularly recorded potentials suggest that they may represent complex summated postsynaptic potentials (PSP) that are predominantly excitatory in the superficial regions of the cerebral explants and inhibitory in the deeper zones (Crain, 1966, 1969). They show, moreover, significant similarities to intracellular PSP records obtained from cortical neurons in neonatal kitten cortex (Purpura, 1969).

Still more complex rhythmical oscillatory afterdischarges can be triggered in many cerebral explants. There stereotyped repetitive sequences generally consist of 3 to 12 large, diphasic

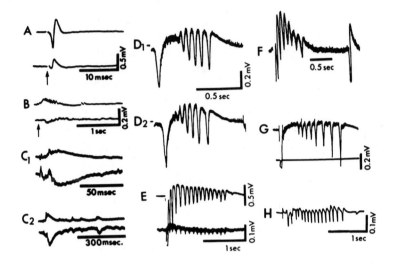

**Figure 1.** *Left section:* Development of complex evoked responses and oscillatory afterdischarges in cultured cerebral cortex tissue, during first 2 weeks after explantation from 1-day-old mouse. *A:* 3 days *in vitro.* Simultaneous records showing simple spikes evoked, at "cortical depths" (see *right section*) of 200 $\mu$ (upper sweep) and 400 $\mu$ by stimulus applied near subcortical edge of explant (about 300 $\mu$ from original cortical surface). *B:* Early signs of complex response patterns recorded, at much slower sweep rate, in same culture and at same electrode loci as in *A.* Long-duration negativity arises gradually with a latency of about 100 msec after the early superficial spike *(upper sweep);* also note long-duration positivity which develops with a still longer latency after early deep spike *(lower sweep).* Arrow indicates onset of dual stimuli spaced 50 msec apart. Note that the second pair of stimuli, applied 1 sec after first pair, is ineffective. $C_1$: 10 days *in vitro.* Simultaneous records of characteristic evoked potentials at "cortical depths" of 250 $\mu$ *(upper sweep)* and 650 $\mu$ following single stimulus applied at depth of 700 $\mu$. Note 60-msec negative evoked response in superficial region and positive response in deep zone which is similar, but of longer duration and greater latency. $C_2$: Same as $C_1$, but at slower sweep rate. Note that small amplitude repetitive potentials at 10 to 20 per sec follow primary responses at both sites and are also of opposite polarities. *D–G:* 2 to 6 weeks *in vitro.* Repetitive oscillatory afterdischarges evoked in four mouse cerebral explants by single stimulus

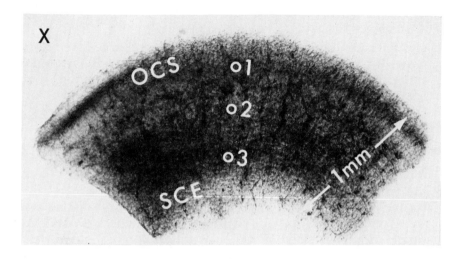

applied several hundred micra from recording site. *Lower record* in *E* shows simultaneous recording from another region of explant (800 $\mu$ away). Note variation in latency of onset of repetitive discharge following initial, positive evoked potential ($D_{1,2}$). *H:* Characteristic repetitive afterdischarge evoked in cerebral cortical slab in 5-day-old kitten, 3 days after neuronal isolation *in situ.* Note similarity between this response pattern and those obtained from cerebral explants (*A* to *G:* Crain, 1964; *H:* Purpura and Housepian, 1961).*Right section:* Photomicrograph of freshly prepared explant of neonatal mouse cerebral cortex (ca. 0.5 mm thick). *OCS:* Original cortical surface; *SCE:* subcortical edge. The tissue has assumed the characteristic crescent shape which it generally maintains for months *in vitro* (Bornstein, 1964). Focal recording electrodes were often positioned, in contact with the tissue, at 1 and 2, and a cathodal stimulating lead placed at 3. Indifferent electrodes were located in fluid near each active electrode. Distance of locus from OCS is referred to as "cortical depth" (Crain, 1964).

*Note:* In this and subsequent figures, time and amplitude calibrations apply to all succeeding records *until otherwise noted;* upward deflection indicates negativity at active recording electrode; all recordings were made with 5 $\mu$ saline-filled or 25 $\mu$ Ag-core pipettes, and electric stimuli were applied via 10 $\mu$ saline-filled pipettes; stimuli were 0.1 to 0.3 msec in duration and their onset is generally indicated, where necessary, by signals below recordings.

potentials, each lasting 25 to 50 msec and occurring at rates of 5 to 15 per sec (Figs. 1B, 1C$_2$, 1D–G; 2A$_{5,6}$). Recordings at multiple sites indicate that these repetitive discharges are highly synchronized over large areas of the explant and may occur spontaneously as well as in response to local stimulation of a few neurons, or even of a single neurite which has grown out from the edge of the explant. Analyses of the spontaneous discharge patterns in these and other types of cultured CNS tissues indicate that "pacemaker" neurons may generate spikes sporadically or rhythmically; these spontaneous impulses can then trigger widespread network discharges depending upon the excitability threshold of the latter system (Corner and Crain, 1969, 1972). These rhythmic oscillatory discharges show remarkable similarity to repetitive sequences evoked by single stimuli in slabs of neonatal kitten cerebral neocortex studied several days after chronic neuronal isolation (Fig. 1H; Purpura and Housepian, 1961a; Purpura, 1969). Although these complex discharges in cerebral slabs *in situ* and *in vitro* show marked hyperexcitability properties, the most significant point is the mimicry displayed by the cultured tissues of intricate bioelectrical patterns characteristic of organized cerebral cortex *in situ*.

The electrophysiological studies of mammalian cerebral explants during maturation in culture demonstrate the intrinsic capacity of these CNS tissues to organize complex synaptic networks after complete isolation *in vitro*. Correlative electron microscopic observations of these explanted tissues before and after development of complex bioelectrical discharge patterns indicate a paucity or absence of synaptic junctions at explantation and an abundance of synapses by the end of the 1st week *in vitro* (Pappas, 1966; Model et al., 1971). An even more dramatic demonstration of the self-organizing properties of cerebral neurons has recently been made with cultures of completely dissociated fetal mouse cerebral cortex, brain stem, and spinal cord cells, during reaggregation and the randomly dispersed neurons *in vitro* (Crain and Bornstein, 1972). After 2 to 4 weeks *in vitro*, complex repetitive spike discharges have been recorded, spontaneously as well as in response to electrical stimuli, from dozens of discrete neuronal clusters which had become attached to the collagen-coated cover glass over an area of about 1 cm$^2$, and appeared to be

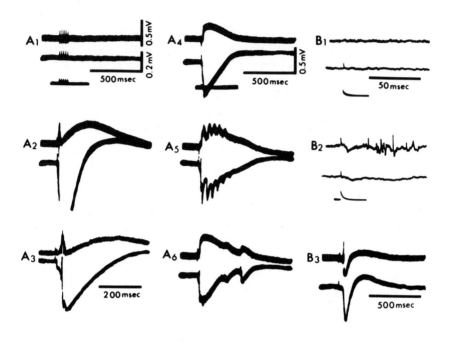

**Figure 2.** Absence of bioelectrical activity in 17-day fetal mouse cerebral neocortex explants during chronic (1-month) exposure to xylocaine (50 $\mu$g per ml) and rapid recovery in normal medium. $A_1$: No responses are evoked while explant is still in culture medium containing xylocaine, even with repetitive stimuli, at high intensity. $A_2$: After transfer to *simple* physiological salt solution (BSS) still containing xylocaine at 50 $\mu$g per ml, *first* stimulus triggers characteristic cerebral evoked potential. Note long duration, large amplitude, and polarity differences (i.e., negative near original cortical surface, *upper sweep;* initially positive at "deeper" cortical site, *lower sweep*). $A_{3,4}$: Similar responses after second and later stimuli. $A_{5,6}$: After transfer to normal medium, responses are still more complex and longer in duration. $B_1$: Absence of responses in another cerebral explant under same conditions as in $A_1$. $B_2$: Bursts of spikes evoked by single stimulus about 2 minutes after transfer to normal medium, following acute exposure to xylocaine at 200 $\mu$g per ml. $B_3$: Characteristic "slow-wave" evoked potentials appear about 1 minute later (Crain et al., 1968a).

connected to one another via complex neuritic bridges. Larger clusters containing more than 20 cells also showed characteristic negative slow waves in association with the spike barrages. The amplitudes of these potentials and the duration and complexity of the discharge sequences were greatly enhanced after introduction of strychnine ($10^{-5}$ M) and blocked by $Mg^{++}$ (5 mM). Furthermore, the spontaneous and evoked activities in the clusters were often clearly synchronized, even between neurons separated by distances greater than 3 mm (with variable latencies reflecting conduction and synaptic delays). Thus, even after complete cellular dispersion, mammalian CNS neurons not only can form synaptic connections following reaggregation in culture, but can also organize into functional synaptic networks with complex properties suggesting involvement of inhibitory as well as excitatory mechanisms.

The possible role of functional neuronal activity on early CNS development has been studied in this model system by chronic exposure of fetal mouse cerebral explants to media containing xylocaine or other chemical agents, at concentrations sufficient to block all nerve impulses during the entire period *in vitro* (Crain et al., 1968a). The neurons in these drugged cultures continued, nevertheless, to develop organized synaptic networks as in normal media, and no morphological deficits could be detected after weeks of exposure, even at the electron microscope level (Model et al., 1971). Furthermore, within minutes after removing the blocking agent from the bathing fluid, the first electrical stimulus applied to such a virginal explant often evoked a complex bioelectric response similar to those seen in mature control explants (Fig. 2). The similarity of these responses to patterns characteristic of organized multisynaptic networks *in situ* suggests that ontogenetic development of some types of complex interneuronal CNS functions may be programmed to occur independent of prior bioelectrical excitation of the cellular elements which make up the system. Furthermore, after endogenous formation of such a neuronal cell assembly in culture, it can be maintained in a quiescent state for at least several weeks yet remain organized with characteristic bioelectrical excitability. Isolated CNS explants provide, therefore, a favorable test object for further studies of the characteristic property of "forward reference" which has been shown, by Coghill (1929) and others, to be of fundamental significance in the development of the nervous system.

These studies of cultured CNS tissues have emphasized that development of many organotypic structures and functions appears to be so tightly coupled to genetic factors that the explants continue to organize in rather stereotyped fashion despite wide variations in environmental conditions. Attempts are now under way to detect more subtle plastic properties of these cultured neural networks which may well be highly dependent upon specific environmental factors. Long term changes in excitability or in bioelectrical discharge patterns would be useful quantitative indicators of such plastic alterations which might be produced by sustained application of electrical stimuli to the CNS explants, especially during critical developmental stages. Attempts to detect developmental alterations by introduction of electrical or chemical gradients critically localized with respect to individual cells within the CNS cultures would also be of great interest. Quantitative experiments of these types are difficult to carry out in the conventional micrurgical chambers which have been generally used for acute microelectrode studies of cultured neurons (Crain, 1966, 1973b). Dr. Crain and his associates have developed, therefore, a radically new technique which permits incorporation of a group of miniaturized, magnetically coupled micromanipulators, along with microelectrodes, inside a gas-tight culture chamber under conditions which still permit convenient *external* control of the manipulators for precise positioning, in three dimensions, at high magnification (Crain and Baer, 1969; Crain 1970b, 1973b). Sterile assembly of the components of this sealed recording chamber is feasible and should provide a valuable method for long term microelectrophysiological and other micrurgical studies on individual cultured neurons, during days or weeks of experimental manipulation, in relation to plasticity phenomena and cellular mechanisms associated with memory and learning (see also Bullock, 1967, and Burns, 1968).

In Dr. Crain's view, chronic extracellular recordings of cultured CNS tissues will also provide a valuable foundation for planning more sophisticated intracellular analyses of the membrane potentials of specific neurons in relation to complex network discharges (Zipser et al., 1973). Without such routine indicators of bioelectrical activity in CNS cultures, a great deal of time and effort may be wasted in preparation for elaborate biophysical or biochemical studies on tissues which have actually failed to develop organotypic functions under a particular set of culture conditions. Tissue culture techniques are still not sufficiently standardized in regard to development of complex CNS networks with characteristic synaptic functions, and microscopic observations of the living cultures are not yet adequate to evaluate the integrity of these interneuronal relationships. Dr. Crain warned that this is especially important to keep in mind in evaluating the functional significance of biochemical and cytological properties of cultured CNS tissues studied without correlative bioelectrical tests on the same specimens. There are often serious variations between CNS cultures prepared under "standard" conditions even in a well established laboratory, so that inferences about the functional integrity of *particular* explants based on bioelectrical studies of this type of culture in another laboratory are, generally, unwarranted extrapolations.

Even under "optimal" culture conditions, CNS explants will generally develop some structural and functional deficits or abnormalities relative to their *in situ* counterparts. Isolation of these small fragments of CNS tissue from their normal connections with other neurons will undoubtedly lead to alterations, at least, in neuronal excitability (Crain, 1969). Surgical isolation may, moreover, selectively damage or eliminate those types of neurons in a CNS explant which are more sensitive to mechanical trauma or to chemical deficiencies in the culture medium. Furthermore, even if synapses do form under a particular set of conditions *in vitro,* the resulting network may be significantly unbalanced regarding normal excitatory and inhibitory components; e.g., abnormal shifts toward inhibitory synaptic dominance may develop in older CNS explants (Crain, 1969). For interdisciplinary studies, therefore, the burden of proof rests upon the investigator to determine the specific functional properties of each group of cultured CNS tissues under the particular set of culture conditions involved. These direct electrophysiological studies will provide, then, a firm foundation for using the cultures as an experimental model system, recognizing fully the degree to which the cultured tissues conform or deviate from their *in situ* counterparts.

Some of the deficits produced in cultured CNS tissues as a result of isolation from other parts of the nervous system may be clarified by pairing a given CNS explant with various other central or peripheral neural (or related) tissues. Apposition of fetal mouse cerebral cortex explants, for example, with spinal cord or brain stem tissues has led to development *in vitro* of functional neuritic connections between the different types of tissues; and sustained excitability changes in cerebral explants appear to have occurred in some cases (Crain et al., 1968b). Trophic interactions between neurons in CNS explants are evidently involved in the development and maintenance of organized synaptic networks in long term cultures (see discussion by Crain in Guth and Windle, 1970). Demonstration of organotypic development of CNS tissues during chronic exposure to xylocaine provides a foundation for further characterization of these neurotrophic factors (Crain et al., 1968a), and similar studies are also being carried out in the somewhat simpler system consisting of paired spinal cord and skeletal muscle explants (Crain, 1970c; Crain et al., 1970; Peterson and Crain, 1970, 1972).

Many of these cultured CNS tissues provide useful model systems for studies of disturbances of brain maturation (Crain, 1969, 1972) as well as for analyses of normal development. Metabolic inhibitors, as well as selective pharmacological, immunological, and other agents can be incorporated into the culture medium to produce structural or functional abnormalities over and above those inherent in the trauma of explantation and the limitations of the culture environment. Hemicholinium-3, for example, appears to produce selective interference in the development of neuromuscular relationships, as well as of some types of neurons, in coupled spinal cord-skeletal muscle explants (Crain and Peterson, 1971). This is in contrast to the absence of any detectable structural effects of much higher concentrations of xylocaine on interneuronal relations in CNS cultures (Crain et al., 1968a). Chronic exposure to immunological agents which may selectively inactivate functionally significant sites on neuronal or glial membranes is another powerful approach which is already being applied to developmental studies with CNS cultures. It has been demonstrated recently, for example, that although fetal CNS explants exposed continuously since explantation to low concentrations of serum from animals with experimental allergic encephalomyelitis are thereby prevented from myelinating (Bornstein and Raine, 1970), organotypic synaptic networks still continue to develop, and these completely unmyelinated CNS tissues show characteristic bioelectrical discharges after weeks or months *in vitro* (Bornstein and Crain, 1971). These studies set limits to speculations regarding the possible role of myelination in relation to functional maturation of the CNS *in situ*.

Regarding the relevance of CNS tissue culture models for problems in mental retardation, Dr. Crain believes experimental techniques are probably at too primitive a stage to permit significant evaluation and prediction of the extent to which such application will be feasible. Analyses of the capacities of CNS explants to carry out more complex plastic functions related to memory and learning (e.g., habituation and conditioning) need to be made (Crain 1973a, b) as a guide to formulating experiments with greater relevance to processes associated with mental retardation.

# Biochemical Approaches to the Study of CNS Tissue Cultures as a Model of Brain Development

G. Lehrer

The development of the explantation technique on the collagen-coated cover slip described by Dr. Bornstein, as well as his demonstration of good myelin formation in CNS cultures, has made it possible to examine a number of biochemical parameters of cultured tissues. One question that has been raised concerns the extent to which the culture is a true model of the brain as it develops *in vivo*. The foregoing functional studies summarized by Dr. Crain clearly demonstrate that CNS cultures are capable of exhibiting a variety of complex electrical activities that indicate their functional integrity. Another approach to the question has been taken by Dr. Lehrer, who described his biochemical studies carried out with the aid of the techniques developed by Lowry.

Dr. Lehrer has shown that there is an essential similarity in the time course of development of various enzymes when rodent cerebellar tissues are examined *in vitro* and *in vivo*. Hexokinase increases to close to adult levels by the 9th day both *in vivo* and in the cultures. Similarly, myelination in the cultures and *in vivo* becomes observable by about the 8th or 9th day. Glucose consumption, lactic dehydrogenase, and malic dehydrogenase (a Krebs cycle enzyme) also increase during this period. The last apparently does not increase as much in the cultures as *in vivo*.

Observations on glucose 6-phosphate dehydrogenase

have been of special interest. This enzyme is a triphosphopyridine nucleotide (TPN)-dependent enzyme of the pentose phosphate shunt. It serves to reduce TPN, a pyridine nucleotide which is primarily concerned with synthetic processes in the cell, particularly the final steps in lipid synthesis (long chain fatty acids and cholesterol). It serves as the principal reducing agent in these synthetic pathways. The fact that glucose 6-phosphate dehydrogenase exhibits a peak *in vivo* at about the 10th postnatal day signifies a great need at this time for reducing equivalents for synthetic purposes. The major function of the pentose phosphate shunt around the 10th day in the rodent brain seems to be to supply these reducing equivalents. The enzyme also supplies pentose for nucleic acid synthesis. However, nucleic acid synthesis occurs earlier in development as well. Furthermore, the relatively small amounts of pentose required for this synthesis are far from the turnover capacity of the pentose phosphate shunt.

Another interesting enzyme is TPN-dependent isocitrate dehydrogenase, which continuously decreases during postnatal development *in vivo*. In tissue culture, however, it is at high levels when the tissue is initially explanted and does not decrease. This indicates a difference between the culture and the *in vivo* system and suggests that some processes which occur in the immature brain and are turned off during *in vivo* maturation continue to operate in culture tissue.

The enzyme β-glucuronidase, which is high during development *in vivo,* goes to markedly high levels in cultures. This is undoubtedly related to activity of lysosomal enzymes in macrophages which appear in older cultures in considerable numbers. Macrophages appear to be much more active in cerebellar cultures than in cerebral cultures.

Although many enzyme changes occur in parallel in mouse cerebellum and cerebrum cultures, this is not true for glucose 6-phosphate dehydrogenase. The cerebral cortex is more mature at birth in the mouse than the cerebellar cortex. A decline in glucose 6-phosphate dehydrogenase occurs *in vivo*, whereas in the cultures there is a marked rise. Isocitric dehydrogenase shows early parallels in the culture and *in vivo* but remains at much higher levels in the culture than in the intact brain, again supporting the view that the culture remains more immature, at least biochemically.

The foregoing studies have suggested additional questions to Dr. Lehrer, such as: What are the environmental factors that influence development on an enzymatic level? Comparison of lactic dehydrogenase isoenzymes shows a predominance of the M type of lactic dehydrogenase early in development, whereas later the H components predominate, contributing most of the increase in lactic dehydrogenase activity. Enzyme induction can be seen in the cultures. In these studies the explant is a piece of cortex in which the surface and depth of the original cortical layers from the anterior portion of the cerebral hemisphere are represented in the surface of the slice, both in the portion which lies against the cover slip and in that exposed to the medium. Whereas *in vivo* gradients of metabolic substrates and oxygen occur from capillary to tissue, in the culture these substances must diffuse into the fragment from the medium, thus establishing new and predictable gradients. If samples are taken for analysis perpendicular to the surface of the culture, both the portion exposed to the medium and the part against the cover slip are from the same original layer of cortex. Thus both should have equal potential with respect to the normal development from the surface downward. The two portions are then analyzed separately (Table I). "Top" is the portion nearest to the medium and "bottom" is the portion farthest from the medium. For hexokinase there is no essential difference, although there is an increase with age (as was shown before) both at the depth and at the surface. The same is true for malic dehydrogenase. However, lactic dehydrogenase, which is equal at the time of

**Table I.** Mouse cerebrum tissue cultures M-129*

| Days in Vitro | | HK | LDH | MDH |
|---|---|---|---|---|
| 0 | Top | $1.94 \pm 0.33$ | $38.0 \pm 2.3$ | $54.3 \pm 8.4$ |
| | Bottom | $2.15 \pm 0.06$ | $37.2 \pm 1.4$ | $61.3 \pm 9.0$ |
| 7 | Top | $2.85 \pm 0.46$ | $35.5 \pm 0.8$ | $95.6 \pm 2.6$ |
| | Bottom | $2.35 \pm 0.34$ | $49.9 \pm 7.6$ | $98.6 \pm 2.2$ |
| 14 | Top | $3.65 \pm 0.30$ | $36.5 \pm 1.7$ | $96.0 \pm 5.3$ |
| | Bottom | $3.36 \pm 0.42$ | $59.0 \pm 2.5$ | $101.1 \pm 5.0$ |

*Each value represents the mean of eight determinations on each of two sister cultures $\pm$ the standard error of the mean.

explantation, shows a greater increase with age in the depth, as compared to the surface. From electrophoretic studies at 14 days *in vitro*, the depth lactic dehydrogenase now shows preponderance of the M-type, while the H-type predominates on the surface. In essence, the relative anoxia at the depth of the culture has caused induction of a lactic dehydrogenase which is best adapted to function under anoxic conditions. A similar situation occurs in the avascular layers of the retina: lactic dehydrogenase also increases in the areas most remote from the blood supply and the lactic acid concentration increases concomitantly. The high levels of lactic dehydrogenase have increased proportions of M-type in relation to H-type isoenzymes.

According to Dr. Lehrer, it is well known that brain glucose metabolism is quite high and that in the immature brain glucose consumption is considerably lower. Several of the developmental parameters of brain glucose metabolism have been demonstrated in cultures, perhaps better than in other systems.

Early studies utilized roller tubes containing relatively large amounts of medium and three cover slips with explanted cerebellum on them, in order to minimize effects of possible evaporation and consequent volume changes. In this crude system, Dr. Lehrer could show some differences which depended upon the composition of the medium and the culture

**Table II.** Glucose metabolism in mature cultures*

| | Gluscose Consumption, MKH | Lactate Production, MKH | Pyruvate Production, mMKH | Glucose NET,† MKH | Glucose EXC.,‡ MKH | Culture Dry Weight, μg |
|---|---|---|---|---|---|---|
| 100 mg% GLU, no TPP | 0.547 (0.127) | 0.933 (0.180) | 42.9 (5.3) | 0.080 | 0.467 | 28.3 |
| 100 mg% GLU, with TPP | 0.451 (0.049) | 0.748 (0.085) | 27.3 (1.6) | 0.077 | 0.374 | 63.6 |
| 600 mg% GLU, no TPP | 0.330 (0.095) | 0.507 (0.061) | 12.7 (2.2) | 0.076 | 0.254 | 77.6 |
| 600 mg% GLU, with TPP | 0.261 (0.028) | 0.336 (0.038) | 4.37 (0.81) | 0.093 | 0.168 | 139.8 |

*Values in parentheses are standard errors of the mean.
†Glucose consumption minus one-half lactate production.
‡Glucose consumption appearing as lactate.

conditions (Table II). When glucose in the medium was 6 mM, glucose consumption, lactate production, and pyruvate production were extremely high. When half of the lactate produced was subtracted from the glucose consumed, a net aerobic glucose consumption was obtained at about 80 millimols per kg per hour, which is very close to that of mature mouse brain. Addition of thiamine pyrophosphate to this medium lowered lactate production and glucose consumption correspondingly. If glucose was increased to the optimal concentration for development of the cultures (40 mM), glucose consumption and lactate production decreased further. When this medium was supplemented with thiamine, glucose consumption and lactate production decreased even further, although lactate production still remained abnormally high.

In general, these cultures did not thrive. Indeed, if one examines the final dry weight of cultures, it becomes apparent that these cultures were rather starved and lost much of their mass in proportion to the deficiency of the medium. However, the net oxidative glucose consumption (that is, the glucose consumption not represented by lactate in the medium) remained remarkably constant.

Because conditions in this rather crude system were far from optimal, attempts were made to measure glucose consumption in cultures in the Maximow slide assembly. However, the amount of medium was at best on the order of 100 $\mu$l. When such a small amount of medium is exposed to the atmosphere, there are marked changes in volume. Even in a moist chamber, unless the vapor pressure in the water supply is very accurately controlled, the culture will either gain or lose water. By adding a trace amount of a metabolically inert concentration standard, tritiated antipyrin, to the culture medium, volume changes could be accounted for and glucose and lactate consumption could be accurately measured.

Table III is a sample of a protocol for an experiment which illustrates the reproducibility and precision of this method of measurement. Table IV summarizes measurements from the 5th to the 8th day, from the 12th to the 15th day, and from the 19th to the 22nd day.

On a dry weight basis, glucose consumption in the immature brain is about half that of the brain when it approaches maturity. By 15 days, most of the enzymes have very closely approached adult levels. Myelination is well on its way, and

**Table III.** Determination of glucose consumption and lactate production in single tissue cultures of rat cerebellum: Typical results and calculations for a single experiment*

| cpm | | Corrected Volume, μl | Dry Weight, μg | Protein, μg | Dry Weight of Protein | Glucose | | | | | | Lactate | | | | | |
|---|---|---|---|---|---|---|---|---|---|---|---|---|---|---|---|---|---|
| 0 | 72hr | 72hr | | | | mM 0 | mM 72hr | Adj. mM 72hr | Δ mM | mMKH DW | mMKH protein | mM 0 | mM 72hr | Adj. mM 72hr | Δ mM | mMKH DW | mMKH protein |
| 2109 | 2633 | 66.4 | 36.3 | 13.2 | 2.75 | 39.9 | 47.0 | 37.6 | 6.6 | 168 | 461 | 0.239 | 0.754 | 0.604 | 0.376 | 9.55 | 26.3 |
| 2158 | 2632 | 65.2 | 30.6 | 12.0 | 2.55 | 41.3 | 51.6 | 42.3 | 3.3 | 99 | 252 | 0.230 | 0.590 | 0.484 | 0.265 | 7.85 | 20.0 |
| 2086 | 2577 | 67.1 | 46.6 | 17.2 | 2.71 | 39.6 | 43.9 | 35.5 | 8.4 | 169 | 455 | 0.255 | 0.742 | 0.601 | 0.357 | 7.15 | 19.4 |
| 2086 | 2626 | 67.1 | 53.9 | 21.0 | 2.57 | 40.8 | 43.0 | 34.2 | 10.9 | 206 | 529 | 0.250 | 0.714 | 0.567 | 0.328 | 5.67 | 14.5 |
| 2115 | 2574 | 66.4 | 52.0 | 20.2 | 2.57 | 41.9 | 43.8 | 36.0 | 10.2 | 175 | 451 | 0.244 | 0.714 | 0.587 | 0.354 | 6.28 | 16.1 |
| 2138 | 2650 | 65.8 | 32.9 | 13.2 | 2.49 | 42.3 | 47.0 | 37.9 | 8.7 | 241 | 603 | 0.244 | 0.707 | 0.571 | 0.338 | 9.44 | 23.5 |
| 2089 | 2572 | 67.1 | 38.6 | 14.9 | 2.59 | 42.0 | 43.0 | 34.9 | 11.4 | 275 | 714 | 0.295 | 0.753 | 0.612 | 0.328 | 7.92 | 20.4 |
| 2154 | 2577 | 65.2 | 48.7 | 15.7 | 3.10 | 40.9 | 39.9 | 33.4 | 11.8 | 220 | 682 | 0.298 | 0.685 | 0.573 | 0.286 | 5.31 | 16.5 |
| 1976 | 2195 | | | | | 41.1 | 49.6 | 44.7 | | | | 0.312 | 0.313 | 0.282 | | | |
| 1996 | 2185 | | | | | 41.9 | 51.2 | 46.8 | | | | 0.297 | 0.335 | 0.306 | | | |
| 2262 | | | | | | 38.5 | | | | | | | | | | | |
| | | | | | 2.66 | | | | | 194 | 518 | | | | | 7.40 | 19.6 |
| | | | | | (0.22) | | | | | (19) | (53) | | | | | (0.57) | (1.4) |

*Corrected volume = [cpm in feeding solution × 62.1 (vol. of F.S.)]/cpm (0 time). Both for glucose and lactate: 72-hr adjusted concentration (mM) = (mM$_{72\,hr}$ × cpm$_0$)/cpm$_{72\,hr}$. Δ(absolute concentration change) = (mM$_0$ − mM$_{72\,adj}$) − (B1$_0$ − B1$_{72\,adj}$). mMKH = [Δ × Corr. vol. (1)]/[dry wt of protein (kg) × time (72 hr)].

**Table IV.** Glucose consumption and lactate production in rat cerebellum tissue cultures, series R-169

| DIV | Glucose | | Lactate | |
|---|---|---|---|---|
| | mMKH DW | mMKH protein | mMKH DW | mMKH protein |
| 5–8 | 101 ± 14 | 269 ± 36 | 1.04 ± 0.27 | 2.7 ± 0.7 |
| 12–15 | 194 ± 19 | 518 ± 53 | 7.40 ± 0.57 | 19.6 ± 1.4 |
| 19–22 | 213 ± 19 | 542 ± 39 | 5.75 ± 1.00 | 14.5 ± 2.1 |

complex polysynaptic pathways are present in the culture, as indicated by Dr. Crain's findings. The values of glucose consumption as shown in the cultures are quite comparable if not identical to those obtained in intact mouse brain during development. They are also quite similar to values of glucose consumption obtained for, say, dorsal root ganglion by quite different methods. The lactate levels are appreciably lower than in the roller tube, and lactate production is close to its level in the living brain. Thus, in the cultures of mouse cerebellum in the Maximow slide assembly, the levels of glucose consumption and lactate production are both very close to those in the maturing brain *in vivo*. These measurements, though apparently cumbersome, turn out to be quite simple, according to Dr. Lehrer. They should provide a useful tool for further studies on the effects of alterations in the environment on brain development.

One environmental alteration of the culture is growth in the presence of diluted experimental allergic encephalomyelitis (EAE) serum. It was noted previously that in this circumstance absolutely no myelin develops, whereas, within 1 or 2 days after the EAE serum is removed and normal serum substituted in the culture medium, the cultures begin to myelinate.

Moreover, although myelination is suppressed in these cultures, there is both ultrastructural and electrophysiological evidence that neurons and polysynaptic pathways develop undisturbed. No mature oligodendroglia are observed, and no myelin is formed as long as the culture is grown in the presence of EAE serum. The obvious question is: What happens to the machinery for myelin production in such a system? Some attempts to answer this question were noted in preliminary studies on the incorporation of inorganic sulfate into cerebroside sulfate, a prominent component of myelin.

At various periods during the life of spinal cord cultures, they were divided into two groups. One group was grown in the presence of 3% EAE serum, while the other was grown in normal feeding solution. Both feeding solutions were also made up to contain radioactive sulfate in very high specific activity. At various times the cultures were exposed for 24 hours to the feeding solution containing radioactive sulfate. They were then washed briefly in balanced salt solution. The specific activity of sulfate in the supernatant medium and the specific activity of brain cerebroside sulfate were determined. Cold cerebroside sulfate was added to the frozen-dried cultures followed by a Folch extraction and chromatography on thin layer plates. The cerebroside sulfate pack was then counted with results shown in Fig. 3.

In the controls grown in normal medium, radioactive sulfate incorporation into cerebroside sulfate showed a marked increase between days 8 and 12 *in vitro*, the time when myelin first appears in the cultures. In the inhibited cultures (i.e., those grown in the presence of EAE serum) by the 6th day there was already marked depression in sulfate incorporation into cerebroside sulfate.

According to Dr. Lehrer, this provides further evidence that much of the cerebroside sulfate synthesized in culture is incorporated into myelin. The inhibited cultures appeared normal in every other respect, and the neurons and the synaptic endings were normal.

In one set of the cultures grown in the presence of EAE serum, the serum was replaced with normal serum on the 14th day. Within the first 24 hours, before any visible evidence of myelin formation, there was a fourfold increase in sulfate incorporation into sulfolipids. At 48 hours, a further rise occurred in incorporation over the inhibited cultures. Over the following 3 days, a very sharp increase was noted in sulfate incorporation into cerebroside sulfate, at a rate paralleling that in the control cultures during myelination. During that period, also, a great increase in myelin could be seen in the cultures.

It is inferred from these studies that in some way the differentiation of machinery in the brain culture which subserves phospholipid incorporation into cerebroside sulfate has been inhibited by the EAE serum. Whether this indicates that maturation of the oligodendrocyte is required (there is a specific enzyme system in the oligodendrocyte concerned with myelin formation) is not yet clear.

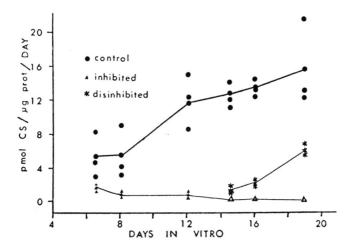

**Figure 3.** The rate of [35]S incorporation into cerebroside sulfate. The results are expressed in nmoles of ([35]S)-sulfate incorporated in cerebroside sulfate during a 24-hour period beginning on the days indicated. Each point represents incorporation by one culture (one cover slip bearing two fragments). The lines were drawn through the mean values for each day. The actual activity of [35]S incorporated per culture ranged: control, 2,000 to 10,000 cpm; inhibited, 75 to 2,000 cpm; and disinhibited, 850 to 4,500 cpm. The amount of ([35]S)-sulfate incorporated was calculated from the determined [35]S specific activity in the feeding medium. All radioactivity measurements were made at the same time; thus, no correction for [35]S decay was necessary. The amount of protein per culture ranged from 16 to 34 μg. (Source: Fry, J. M., Lehrer, G. M., and Bornstein, M. B. 1972. Sulfatide synthesis in CNS tissue culture and its inhibition by EAE serum. Science 175: 192–193.)

As Dr. Lehrer pointed out, cerebroside $\beta$-galactosidase is an enzyme which differentiates or appears in brain at about the same time that mature oligodendrocytes are first seen (Bowen and Radin, 1969). It has been suggested that this enzyme may be specific for the oligodendrocyte. Dr. Lehrer's studies in progress are concerned with determining whether this enzyme is induced at myelination or is prevented from being induced by the EAE serum.

The biochemical studies summarized by Dr. Lehrer indicate an approach using tissue culture material which can provide direct information on differentiation of the oligodendrocyte and the mechanisms of myelin formation in the brain. He believes that the importance of this problem in developmental neurobiology cannot be overemphasized.

# Problems in Culture Analysis of Neurological Mutant Disorders

M. Wolf

Apart from the usefulness of tissue culture techniques for investigating problems of morphophysiological and biochemical development, tissue culture methodology makes possible the experimental analysis of many genetic defects, as reported by Dr. Wolf.

The achievement of histoarchitectonic differentiation in long term "organotypic" cultures of embryonic brain fragments (Bornstein and Murray, 1958; Wolf, 1964, 1970; Wolf and Dubois-Dalcq, 1970) opens the door to using such organotypic cultures for the analysis of those defective genes which alter brain histoarchitectonics *in situ* (Sidman, Green, and Appel, 1965). To illustrate the pitfalls of such experiments, four studies of mutant mice were reviewed by Dr. Wolf.

*Jimpy*, a sex-linked recessive lethal gene, produces uniform severe CNS myelin deficiency, with tremor, convulsions, and death shortly after weaning (Sidman, Dickie, and Appel, 1964). Cultures of mouse cerebellum will produce abundant myelin but must be started from 0- to 2-day-old mice, 10 to 12 days before clinical or anatomical expression of the disease. This problem was overcome (Wolf and Holden, 1969) by the use of mice in which *Tabby*, a sex-linked semidominant gene, served as a marker for affected, heterozygous, and normal newborns. The jimpy disease is reproduced *in vitro*. Jimpy cultures have either very scanty myelin or none at all but are normal in neuronal and axonal architecture, while all types of controls are normal in both neuron and myelin development.

Combined cultures of jimpy and normal brains suggest that the gene may influence a cell-bound rather than a diffusible mechanism. Serial observations of jimpy cultures indicate that the defect probably occurs in myelin lipid biosynthesis, rather than involving destruction of fully formed myelin sheaths, as was previously thought.

*Quaking,* an autosomal recessive gene on the 9th linkage group, also produces severe CNS myelin deficiency, tremor, and convulsion, presumably by a different mechanism than jimpy (Sidman, Dickie, and Appel, 1964). The myelin deficiency is somewhat less severe than jimpy's but would be readily recognized in culture were it expressed in the same way. No marker gene is available, but affected animals survive longer than those with jimpy, and the females can be bred. Thus, affected females were bred to heterozygous males to obtain litters which would contain on the average 50% affected and 50% heterozygous offspring. When such litters were used for culture, about 50% of the animals produced well myelinated cultures, while the other 50% produced cultures with little or no myelin. However, these cultures were deficient, not only in myelin, but also in large neurons and long axons. This did not resemble the diseased quaking brain *in situ* but rather resembled cultures which have "failed to thrive" for myriad unknown reasons. Since it was not known whether the deficient cultures were from quaking animals, it could not be decided whether their deficiency represented a pleiotropic effect of the quaking gene. Perhaps some other gene in the non-inbred stock originally carrying quaking was responsible. However, the same result was obtained 2 years later from a congenic subline of inbred C57BL/6J mice, the standard for culture work in Dr. Wolf's laboratory, to which the quaking gene had been transplanted by outcross-intercross matings. The same result was even obtained from crosses of heterozygous C57BL/6J quaking males to *normal* females. Thus, according to Dr. Wolf, the culture results are uninterpretable. They may conceivably be due to some coincident abnormality in the closely linked, complicated T locus. In this light, it is interesting that homozygous quaking males are sterile because of defects in spermatogenesis (Bennett, Gall, Southard, and Sidman, 1971).

*Dilute-lethal,* an autosomal recessive gene, produces a deficiency of phenylalanine hydroxylase leading to pigment dilution, neurological incapacitation, and early death. The disease is similar, though not in every respect, to human phenylketonuria, and myelin degeneration has been reported as a morphological finding in both the mouse and human diseases. An inbred strain of mice carrying dilute-lethal and the recessive marker gene *short-ears* in repulsion was used for culture. Short-eared homozygotes have a defective xiphisternum recognized at birth. Glycerol-cleared whole mounts of skin, after 2 to 3 days of incubation, clearly show the difference between the pigment granule distribution of dilute-lethal homozygotes and normal mice. Animals normal by both criteria were presumed to be heterozygous at both loci. Dilute-lethal, heterozygous, and normal cultures from this strain were all as heavily myelinated, well differentiated, and long lived as any in the experience of Dr. Wolf's laboratory. They survived for at least 106 days, whereas no dilute-lethal mouse has yet survived 50 days even with special care. However, reexamination of the histopathology of dilute-lethal mouse and the phenylketonuric human brains cast doubt on the previous reports of myelin destruction. Interpretation of the human material was complicated by malnutrition, repeated convulsions with consequent trauma and anoxia, and other intercurrent disease. The first two factors apply with equal force to the mouse material which, furthermore, has previously been examined by the Marchi method for degenerating myelin, now generally abandoned as unreliable. Quantitative comparison (Kemper and Jacobson, unpublished studies) of dilute-lethal with normal siblings revealed, indeed, retarded development of myelin and of the synaptic neuropil. However, similar retardation was obtained in mice which were neurologically normal but were undersized for nonspecific nutritional or genetic reasons. Dr. Wolf and his colleagues have come to doubt that dilute-lethal produces any primary defect in brain morphology. There is surely none that can be recognized and studied in the tissue culture setting.          ·

By contrast, the morphological defect produced by the recessive gene *nervous* should be readily identifiable in culture. Nervous mice lose most of their cerebellar Purkinje cells by degeneration between 3 and 6 weeks of age. Cultures from the cerebellar hemispheres, where few Purkinje cells survive, can be compared with cultures from the vermis, where more are spared. Homozygous animals will breed, providing litters with 100% affected animals. The dilemma, as noted by Dr. Wolf, is that the nervous mutation occurred in a subline of the BALB/C inbred strain, and cultures from brains of this strain develop poorly for unknown genetic reasons. The nervous gene has been transferred to a C57BL/6J subline, but on this particular background it produces a much less severe disease, with fewer degenerating cells, which would probably not be recognizable in the culture setting. Until a genetic background is found which permits both adaptation of brain tissue to culture and full expression of the nervous disease, this culture study cannot be carried out.

According to Dr. Wolf, comparison of successful, unsuccessful, and abortive studies helps to define the following prerequisites for the culture analysis of a genetic disorder:

1. A phenotype for which some nonambiguous property can be defined in the culture system;
2. Control over the genotype, with regard to:
    a. Identification of the affected animals at the appropriate stage, often before the disease is expressed;
    b. Exclusion of other genes which may affect either adaptability to culture or the expression of the phenotype in the culture system.

# The Search for Additional Simple Neuronal Systems: The Microtubule and Clonal Neuroblastoma Systems

**M. Shelanski**

Two areas of research in neurobiology have attracted considerable interest in recent years, according to Dr. Shelanski. The first of these is concerned with the neurotubule or microtubule system in which the subcellular organelle may be readily studied and manipulated. The second is concerned with the clonal neuroblastoma system. Some of the salient features of work on these systems have been summarized by Dr. Shelanski.

Microtubules are ubiquitous organelles which are found in most if not all eukaryotic cells. They appear as hollow tubes with a diameter of 240 A and often are very long. In many cases they are organized for special functions, such as forming the spindle fibers of the mitotic spindle, of the axoneme, or of the cilium or flagellum. In the cilium or flagellum the tubules are organized into two central single tubules and nine pairs of joined tubules in a circle around the central pair. Taylor (1965) reasoned that since colchicine blocked mitosis in metaphase, thus causing a loss in the birefringence normally seen along these fibers, it might bind to the subunit of the spindle fibers. His experiments on colchicine effects on cells revealed that, at the concentrations used, colchicine did not block DNA, RNA, or protein synthesis but did bind to an intracellular macromolecule in a semistable manner. The colchicine-binding activities of a number of cells and tissues were studied and correlated roughly with mitotic activity except in the case of brain, which had a low mitotic index but extremely high colchicine-binding levels (Borisy and Taylor, 1967a). This apparent problem was reconciled with the realization that the dendrites and axons of neurons were rich in microtubules. A similar colchicine-binding protein with a sedimentation velocity of 6S and a molecular weight of approximately 100,000 daltons was obtained from the isolated mitotic apparatus (Borisy and Taylor, 1967b). To identify this protein with the microtubules, the central pair of sperm flagellum tubules was isolated by low ionic strength dialysis and found to be composed of a single protein which was solubilized as a 6S, 120,000-dalton dimer which bound 1 mole of colchicine and 2 moles of GTP per dimer (Shelanski and Taylor, 1967, 1968). Shortly thereafter, the microtubule subunit protein was purified from brain (Weisenberg, Borisy, and Taylor, 1968).

The microtubule protein is one of the major soluble proteins in the brain. It is rapidly synthesized and turned over with a half-life of 4 days (Feit and Shelanski, unpublished observations). It makes up an astonishing 18% of the soluble protein of the brain and perhaps even more astonishing 28 to 30% of the soluble protein in synapsomes (Feit et al., 1971). Clearly, it is a protein of some importance in the brain.

Starting with the work with colchicine by Peterson, as well as by Wisniewski and Terry (1967) and Bensch and Malawista with vinblastine, it was observed that the treatment of cells and nervous tissue with an antimitotic caused the formation first of fibrils and, in the case of vinblastine, of crystals (Bensch and Malawista, 1968, 1969).

Drs. Shelanski and Marantz decided to study formation of crystals in vitro. Surprisingly, it was found that, when vinblastine was added to a solution of purified microtubule protein, all of the protein and the colchicine-binding activity precipitated. Vinblastine was then tried with 100,000 g of supernatant from a variety of tissues and from brain with the same result: a precipitate which gave one band in electrophoresis that included all the colchicine-binding activity. The structure of the precipitate was very similar to the crystals seen in cells treated with vinblastine (Marantz and Shelanski, 1970).

This method gave a rapid 10-minute quantitative

purification for a major, probably structural, protein from the nervous system. It is useful, Dr. Shelanski noted, because the simple biochemical technique does not require the complex procedure of ammonium sulfate fractionating and diethyl-aminoethyl cellulose chromatography.

It was emphasized by Dr. Shelanski that this method, however, must not be applied uncritically. Vinblastine can, in addition to its specific effects, act in synergy with divalent cations to precipitate a wide variety of proteins. Therefore, it is necessary to control carefully magnesium and vinblastine con-centrations as well as the purity of the final product by gel electrophoresis. If these precautions are followed, the vinblas-tine precipitation method provides a useful, quantitative, and rapid purification of tubulin. Unfortunately, the vinblas-tine-precipitated material is in a 28S polymeric form and is not suitable for physicochemical studies which should begin with the native 6S dimeric form.

An interesting application of what has been learned about microtubules, according to Dr. Shelanski, is the study of axon outgrowth in neurons. One of the earliest attempts in the nervous system was that of Daniels (1968), who studied ex-planted trypsinized and dissociated neurons in culture and showed that colchicine would inhibit axon outgrowth. Removal of colchicine permitted outgrowth to continue in a normal manner. This implied that the microtubules were necessary to axon outgrowth, while protein synthesis was not.

Dr. Shelanski noted a parallel to these experiments in experiments on flagellar regeneration which showed that the colchicine would block the outgrowth of the flagellum, a struc-ture which grows out at about the same rate as the axon and, like the axon, is rich in microtubules. In this preparation, too, protein synthesis was not necessary for the outgrowth (Rosen-baum and Carlson, 1969).

To study these phenomena in a more controlled manner, simpler neuronal systems have been sought. One such system, noted above, is the explanted neuronal culture of the type pioneered by Murray and Bornstein. A second type is the more recently introduced neuroblastoma system.

Human neuroblastomas were cultured and shown by Goldstein (1968) to undergo a type of neuronal differentiation with neurite outgrowth. Recently, the C-1300 mouse neuroblastoma, which has been carried in animals for many years at the Jackson Labs, has been used. Cultures are prepared by dissociation followed by cloning. Two clones are currently being used by Dr. Shelanski and his colleagues: Neuro 2A, derived by Ruddle at Yale, and N-18 from Nirenberg's laboratory at the NIH.

The N-18 is of interest, according to Dr. Shelanski, because it will put out processes best in low serum. Sprouting is induced in passage from 10% serum to no serum. As in the case of Daniels' neuroblasts, this sprouting is blocked by colchicine but not by cyclohexamide. To Dr. Shelanski these results add additional support to the hypothesis that microtubule assembly is necessary for axon outgrowth, while protein synthesis is not, at least over short time intervals (Seeds et al., 1970).

It is interesting that such parallels in process extension exist between the neuron and the neuroblastoma. At least some clones of neuroblastoma have excitable membranes and others have various "neuronal" enzymes such as tyrosine hydroxylase and choline acetylase. Not all activities are present in all clones, which may also differ in morphology one from the other. These differences between clones may be great or small.

Dr. Shelanski warned that, on the one hand, investigators seeking a "model" neuron must be wary of these differences. For example, Schubert and Jacob (1970) have reported a clone which would not put out an axon in the absence of protein synthesis under any conditions. Although this is an example of a small difference, there could be very large ones.

On the other hand, as Dr. Shelanski noted, these differences may be exploited. Clones can be used like mutants in bacterial genetics to study control mechanisms. This involves "mating" or hybridizing the two parent strains with Sendai virus or a similar agent and studying the progeny. One can also make hybrids with non-neural cells to attempt to gain a further understanding of neuronal differentiation.

Still, according to Dr. Shelanski, the nagging question remains: Are these really neurons? The answer is not easily given. Division continues in neuroblastoma while adult neurons do not divide. True synapses between neuroblastoma cells have not been observed, but the problem really has not received adequate study. Electron microscopic studies have failed, to this date, to reveal any synaptic vesicles.

The arguments are continuously raised that these systems are abnormal and neoplastic and that results based on them are invalid. More rarely, one hears these cells called "neurons." Both approaches are extreme, in Dr. Shelanski's view. The neuroblastomas and other clonal lines are model systems which in many ways resemble neurons. Thus, neurobiologists may use them to advance the field much in the same way that cell biologists have used cell lines such as HeLa, KB, and L. Finally, many of the lines of neuroblastoma in use today in laboratories are pleuropnemonia-like organisms-(PPLO)-contaminated; they are thus worthless for studies in nucleic acid metabolism, especially RNA. Extreme caution must be exercised to make sure that cultures are PPLO-free.

To determine whether these colchicine effects are related to axon outgrowth, Dr. Shelanski believes that one should investigate the microtubule protein in the axon outgrowth, perhaps using the vinblastine precipitation method. However, when Feit in Dr. Shelanski's laboratory first applied this method to very dilute solutions such as lysed synaptosomal supernatants, the precipitate was small or not pure. Concentration of these solutions was needed to get good precipitate and purity.

In addition, one must be very careful with magnesium concentrations. If magnesium is too high, the vinblastine precipitation brings down other proteins besides tubulin. Thus, the method must be monitored by disc gel electrophoresis or by some other assay.

Attempts have been made to incorporate radioactivity into cell bodies and nerve endings at various times. In collaborative studies with Feit, Dutton, and Barondes, Dr. Shelanski found that 15 minutes after injection of a pulse of leucine into the brain there was a rather extensive incorporation into protein and a large peak on disc gels with a molecular weight about 55,000.

At 90 minutes this peak was even larger, but at 24 hours there was a considerable fall. Some of this activity had left the cell body, via either metabolism or axonal transport.

When the nerve endings were examined, quite the opposite was found. At 15 and 90 minutes, there was very little incorporation at 60,000 m.w., but at 24 hours, there was a huge peak that comigrated with the tubulin peak. This has been taken as evidence of axonal transport of the tubule protein.

One conclusion drawn by Dr. Shelanski from these varied studies is that the tubule protein is transported. It goes down the axon, and colchicine blocks the transport of constituents down the axon. This has been demonstrated by many groups, starting with Kreutzberg. Colchicine appears to be able to block first the fast component of axoplasmic transport and then the slow. Microtubule transport itself is in the slow component. Evidently axoplasmic transport and axon outgrowth are related processes. Certainly, the rates of axon outgrowth and nerve regeneration parallel the rates of axoplasmic transport. Colchicine affects both systems in a similar manner.

In Dr. Shelanski's view, the system of vinblastine precipitation for studying the metabolism and behavior of microtubule protein will be very useful in future studies of axonal metabolism. In this connection he noted reports that secretion in many endocrine cells is blocked by colchicine and vinblastine. This fits nicely with the observation by Feit and Barondes (1970) which shows colchicine binding at the synaptosomal membrane. One can see in such fractions proteins which migrate with the microtubule protein on gel electrophoresis. The neuroblastoma provides a source for studying such a mechanism; large quantities of cells can be grown which can be made to differentiate at will. It also provides systems in which clones can be derived which are the equivalent of mutants. One can obtain a clone with or without tyrosine hydroxylase. Some clones will put out axons in low serum, while others will put out axons in high serum. Perhaps one can find clones resistant to colchicine effects on axon outgrowth.

Hybridization studies and biochemical analyses of these cells should allow the neurobiologist, like the cell biologist before him, to be able to select mutants for appropriate characteristics and study.

# Highlights of General Discussion Following Session I on Simple Neuronal Systems

D. P. Purpura

During the discussion period, the validity of using the neuroblastoma cell as a model for normal nervous tissue was questioned. It was pointed out that the origin of the murine neuroblastoma was unclear; that its morphology *in vitro* bore no resemblance to that of the neuroblastoma *in vivo;* and, finally, that the neuroblastoma is, after all, a tumor cell. These arguments were vigorously challenged by various participants who stressed the important role of cultures of malignant cells such as the HeLa cell in the recent development of concepts in cell biology. It was also noted that the neuroblastoma may be studied with electrophysiological as well as biochemical techniques, and correlations effected between bioelectrical and metabolic properties. There was general agreement that the neuroblastoma system would indeed open up important new areas of neurobiological investigation.

Discussion also focused on the extent to which the use of disaggregated cell systems might provide a means for studying the earliest development of synaptic relations. Several of the speakers commented on results of their current investigations which appear to confirm the value of the method. The problems posed by examining the consequences of failures of disaggregated cells to form their normal synaptic connections were mentioned. It was suggested that this approach to the study of neuronal interactions might profitably lead to understanding the factors required for normal maintenance of synaptic relations in developing and mature neuronal subsystems.

# SESSION II.
# NEUROCHEMISTRY OF BRAIN MATURATION

# Statement of the Problem

W. Norton

It is frequently heard that there is no such discipline as neurochemistry, there is only biochemistry. However one wishes to argue the matter, it is obvious, as Dr. Norton indicated, that the methods most useful in advancing the field are those which are not specific to neurochemistry, but apply to the whole field of biochemistry. For example, subcellular fractionation, with its particular application to the CNS for the isolation of special brain structures; special developments in chromatography, such as gas-liquid and thin-layer chromatography; and tracer techniques, among others, have been the methodological advances in the past 20 years which have proven most useful in neurochemistry.

As noted by Dr. Norton, every neurochemist must of necessity be a developmental neurobiologist. The dramatic changes in all brain parameters during development make it necessary to consider the maturational stages of the brain very carefully when planning and conducting any neurochemical research. These stages are generally divided into the following five major periods: 1) neuronal proliferation and migration; 2) glial proliferation; 3) dendritic growth and synapse formation; 4) myelination; and 5) general growth.

There are two major problems facing the chemist. One is that any particular developmental event does not occur simultaneously in all parts of the brain; the other is that these developmental events overlap each other in time, even in circumscribed brain areas which are rather homogeneous in development.

In Dr. Norton's view, much of the chemist's contribution to the study of brain development has been in the area of mensuration. This analytical approach has been very productive, and the existing methodology is generally excellent. Essentially any chemical constituent can be measured quantitatively by existing techniques, or by methods applying established principles. This statement applies equally to the measurement of chemical constituents or enzymatic activities.

The neurochemist would like to know how these neurochemical parameters correlate with morphological and physiological events during maturation. One hopes to be able to find a "marker": a compound or enzyme which is specific for a particular cell, subcellular fraction, or structure. By following the amount of the marker during development, a semiquantitative idea of the accumulation or change of the structure can be achieved.

Many markers are commonly used; some are quite specific, while others are not. One of the most common is DNA, an excellent marker for cell number since most cells in the CNS are diploid and therefore have the same DNA content. This marker does not, of course, differentiate one cell from another, but it is very useful in determining the total number of cells. It is much more difficult to follow the accumulation of neurons and glial cells separately. The nervous system-specific protein, S-100, is probably a glial marker, but it is not certain whether this is a marker for astrocytes or oligodendrocytes; it probably occurs in both types of glia. Among other nervous system-specific proteins, the 14-3-2 protein is apparently specific for neurons.

The myelin sheath has many markers. Cerebroside is generally considered one of the better ones for following myelin accumulation. The myelin-specific proteins, basic protein and proteolipid protein, are also useful. Recently the enzyme 2', 3-cyclicnucleotide-3'-phosphohydrolase has been found to be myelin-specific and a useful myelin marker. This enzyme also is present in oligodendroglia. It may develop that this enzyme, as well as the enzymes involved in cerebroside synthesis, may be useful markers for the myelin-generating cell.

There are, of course, other markers for various subcellular fractions, i.e., the lysosomal degradative enzymes and mitochondrial enzymes. It is generally agreed that $Na^+$, $K^+$-activated ATPase and 5'-nucleotidase are markers for plasma membranes. Gangliosides have been considered markers for neuronal plasma membranes, more specifically, perhaps, the synaptosome. As investigations become more sophisticated, it is frequently found that the assumed specificity of markers decreases. For example, gangliosides are now found in all CNS cells.

It frequently happens that methodology which was developed for mature brain is found to be inadequate when applied to immature brain. One example can be found in the studies of myelination during development. These studies went through a series of successive refinements as knowledge increased and methodology became more elegant.

Biochemical studies on myelination started with the analysis of whole brain during development. Through such studies it was suggested that cerebroside and sulfatide were myelin markers. The next step was the development of myelin isolation techniques and the extensive analysis of myelin from the adult brain. This work cast some doubt on the specificity of the presumed markers. These isolation techniques were then applied to the developing brain but were eventually recognized as inadequate. Until this realization, the picture was very confused, and there were many conflicting reports concerning the real nature of myelin during development. Did it change in composition? If so, was it considerably different from the adult type or only slightly different? It was necessary to devise new isolation methods which could be applied to all ages of development. Several different forms of myelin exist: the adult form, the immature form, and possibly a membrane which is a precursor of the immature form. Thus myelin is not a constant chemical entity.

These membrane studies were done with existing techniques for lipid assays. In the interim new advances in methodology made it possible to study the proteins as well. Previous studies must be repeated with this advanced methodology.

Since such studies were carried out with myelin isolated from whole brain, they are not definitive. It is now necessary to reexamine myelin from homogeneous areas of brain and cord, where myelination occurs simultaneously in all parts of this particular substructure.

Finally, for such a study, the problem of definition arises. What is myelin? Does one seek a morphological, operational, or chemical definition? For many areas of neurochemistry current methodology probably only permits examination of the first few boxes of a nearly endless nest of boxes.

According to Dr. Norton, myelination is one major developmental stage that the neurochemist has characterized and followed rather well. There are, however, other critical developmental stages that cannot be well characterized at present. For example, there is no good biochemical way of following the elaboration of the dendritic tree; nor can synapse formation be followed adequately. The ratio of neurons to glia in the brain at any age is not known (values in the literature for this ratio differ by a factor of ten in some instances). In addition, the ratio or total number of astrocytes vs. oligodendroglia in a particular sample cannot be defined. Hopefully, the methods currently being developed to separate and isolate neurons and glia will provide the means to obtain much of this basic information.

Dr. Norton pointed out that still other problems probably need conceptual breakthroughs. These are areas where there is a danger of working beyond the technology and therefore of being, at the very least, inefficient. The whole problem of the biochemistry of memory and learning and the basis of intelligence may very well be one of those areas. Even though a number of significant advances have been made, major new concepts are required before this work can proceed much further.

# Biochemical Approaches to the Developing Nervous System

G. McKhann

## MYELIN FORMATION

There have been a number of studies of myelin in terms of its chemical composition, ultrastructural properties, and metabolism of its components, primarily lipids. In Dr. McKhann's laboratory (in conjunction with J. Benjamins, D. Farrell, and M. Guarnieri) the focus has been on three extensions of these previous types of studies.

### The Structure of the Myelin Membrane

Dr. McKhann noted that a crucial question is whether the plasma membrane of the oligodendrocyte has the same composition as that of myelin. In previous approaches, the chemical composition of cells obtained from tumors, such as oligodendrogliomas, was compared with the composition of myelin. The evidence obtained from such studies has been indirect, at best. There are systems, such as the myelinating tissue culture, in which the oligodendrocyte can be seen to change in its over-all morphology as myelination begins. At present there is no system for obtaining oligodendrocytes from cultures in a purified fraction. However, cell separation systems such as those of Dr. Norton may be adapted to this problem. An alternate approach is to use antibodies to components of myelin and note whether these antibodies also bind to or interact with the plasma cell membrane of the oligodendrocyte. Studies of this type are in progress using antibodies prepared to basic protein, galactocerebroside, and sulfatide.

Use of antibodies to study the three-dimensional structure of a membrane has been successful in the study of the mitochondrial membrane. This approach is being adapted in Dr. McKhann's laboratory to the study of myelin and, hopefully, to the plasma cell membrane of the oligodendrocyte. These workers believe that the enzyme or antibody which interacts with a component of the membrane will interact only if active chemical groups are exposed on the surface of the membrane. For example, in mature myelin, basic protein appears to be exposed and approachable by an antibody to this protein, while certain phospholipids are only exposed to a phospholipase when the myelin is altered by freezing and thawing or by treatment with a proteolytic enzyme.

These studies are being continued both in intact myelin and in myelinating tissue cultures to see if this approach can provide some leads as to the structure of the membrane of the oligodendrocyte and its changes as myelination progresses.

### Site of Synthesis of Myelin

When myelination takes place, there is a rapid increase in synthesis of protein and lipid components of myelin. Somehow these components must be assembled in an integrated unit and introduced into the membrane. Previous studies in Dr. McKhann's laboratory have suggested that one lipid component, sulfatide, is synthesized by the endoplasmic reticulum and transported through the cytoplasm, attached to a soluble lipoprotein, and introduced into the final myelin membrane. Recent evidence suggests that phospholipids are not handled in a similar fashion. As an extension of these studies, the effects on this system of protein synthesis inhibitors have been analyzed. Puromycin, which can effectively block the introduction of a labelled amino acid into both total protein and myelin protein, has much less effect on the introduction of an appropriate label into a particular lipid. Despite the fact that all new protein synthesis is inhibited, the introduction of lipids into myelin continues to take place. In addition, lipid introduced into myelin appears to be as stable as those lipids introduced into myelin in control animals. This series of observations is being continued, but one possible interpretation at present is that lipids are attached to some kind of template protein which is already present before the period of protein inhibition. Sequential studies of the effects of protein inhibitors are now in progress in Dr. McKhann's laboratory.

## Premyelin Membrane

Members of Dr. McKhann's group, like others, have been interested in identifying stages in the formation of myelin in which some kind of premyelin membrane could exist. One might postulate, however, that this premyelin membrane might be particularly enriched in the specific myelin proteins but not yet have its full complement of myelin lipids. Recently, using density gradient centrifugation techniques, several myelin-like bands have been obtained by McKhann and his co-workers from animals which are actively myelinating. The properties of these particular myelin-like fractions are now under investigation.

## Systems for Studying Myelin Formation

The formation of myelin can be studied under a number of different conditions. One can use a small animal in which myelinization takes place in an explosive fashion. Under these circumstances, however, it is difficult to study any particular anatomical tract. One has to deal with the whole brain. Myelinating tissue cultures have the advantage that they can be used in a more synchronous fashion and one can correlate morphological happenings with what one is studying. Myelinating tissue cultures have been used in Dr. McKhann's laboratory to study the introduction of certain lipids into myelin. For these studies carrier myelin has been added to aid in isolation. Using this technique, instead of having to pool 50 to 100 cultures, each weighing 0.5 mg, one can take only 2 or 3 cultures and add them to a homogenate from whole brain. If myelin has been isolated, then the only labelled myelin must come from the cultures. Utilizing carrier myelin in this way may greatly facilitate use of the culture system for metabolic experiments.

The culture system can be used for the study of the onset of myelin formation, as has been discussed by Dr. Bornstein, and also for the experimental study of demyelinating factors, as has been done by Drs. Bornstein and Lehrer. An extension of this approach is the type of investigation which Dr. McKhann's laboratory is carrying out in collaboration with Dr.

Radin of the University of Michigan. In these studies, analogues of cerebroside which may block either the synthesis or degradation of cerebroside are added to actively myelinating cultures or those which have already myelinated. It is thus possible to see whether altering the metabolism of a specific component of myelin has a direct effect on myelin formation or maintenance. Preliminary observations show that this approach is feasible and that specific compounds appear to affect the maintenance of myelin.

**Other Questions Regarding Myelin and Its Study**

In Dr. McKhann's view, in a number of areas satisfactory techniques are unavailable to answer the essential questions. For example, the mechanism of isolating myelin for biochemical studies is not completely satisfactory. The repeated washing, osmotic shock, and centrifugation techniques result in a product which may be skewed toward a stable inert membrane from which more active parts of the myelin fraction have been torn away. Thus one may get a very biased view of the metabolic inertness of myelin or of its chemical composition. According to Dr. McKhann, one possible approach to this problem would be some kind of membrane electrophoresis, taking advantage of the charge on the myelin membrane. He believes that these techniques have not been satisfactorily tried; he and his co-workers have no real personal experience with them.

A second problem concerns the desire to study myelin at various times in its development. Although the tissue culture system may be the best for this, even tissue cultures are not entirely synchronous in their patterns and rates of myelin formation. However, the proper development of membrane probes may allow small amounts of myelin to be studied in an intact state to follow the sequential changes in composition.

Finally, there is no conclusive evidence that one can alter the pattern of myelin formation in either an *in vivo* or *in vitro* situation. Attempts with altered nutrition or hypothyroidism have suggested that the time of onset of myelin formation is unchanged although the rate of myelinization is altered. Dr. McKhann believes that it will be of interest if the curve of myelin formation can be shifted to an earlier or later time. The closest approach to this is Dr. Bornstein's system in which myelinating cultures are held by dilute concentrations of serum from animals with allergic encephalomyelitis.

## THE STUDY OF MODELS OF HUMAN DISEASES

Dr. McKhann observed that there are a number of diseases in which development of the human nervous system is altered. Some of these are storage diseases in which abnormal amounts of a normal substance accumulate in neurons, as in Tay-Sachs disease or $GM_1$ gangliosidosis. In contrast, the leukodystrophies are characterized by defects in myelin metabolism in which a substance such as galactocerebroside or sulfatide accumulates. In general, such diseases in which lipids accumulate are related to defects in the catabolism of sphingolipids. There are a number of other diseases such as ceroid-lipofuscinosis (Batten-Vogt disease) in which some other material is stored, the nature of which has not yet been established. A far larger group of diseases exists in which there is neuronal degeneration without any evidence of abnormal storage. Perhaps the presenile and senile dementias, with a possible defect in microtubular protein, are an example of the latter type of disease.

To aid investigation of these degenerative diseases, Dr. McKhann believes it would be very helpful to have animal models so that the appearance of the disease, its course, and its possible alternation could all be followed. Dr. McKhann's laboratory recently had the opportunity to study a Siamese cat with an accumulation of ganglioside relating to a deficiency of the $\beta$-galactosidase responsible for the degradation of the $GM_1$ form of ganglioside. This appears to be a direct model of the comparable human disease. Thus at least one model of a human disease involving ganglioside metabolism is now available, permitting some of the questions raised to be explored more productively. Other models exist as well, such as the Cairn terrier with metachromatic leukodystrophy. It is hoped that other models of human diseases will be found so that the comparative pathology and biochemistry can be established and proper experiments devised.

Another approach to this type of degenerative disease, isolating the abnormal neurons, has been tried in Dr.

McKhann's laboratory and also by Menkes in California. In this way one can deal primarily with the abnormal cell without dilution by the more numerous glia cells which may not show any compositional defect. Studies such as these, which are still in their infancy, will require greater attempts to develop neuronal isolation and maintenance in culture.

# Approaches to Studies of the Effects of Malnutrition on Brain Development

**M. Winick**

The search for suitable "markers" in experimental studies of brain development has led several workers to employ DNA content as a marker for the number of cells in the mammalian brain. Work by Dr. Winick has focused on the usefulness of this and other related methods in examining the effect of malnutrition on brain growth and development.

In describing his studies, Dr. Winick indicated that, although the DNA marker technique has been in vogue for a number of years, it is not specific for differentiating one cell type from another. In certain organs in which cells exhibit a change in ploidy with development, the technique is not valuable as an indicator of cell number. However, in studies of brain cells, some of which have a small amount of ploidy (which does not change with development), the DNA marker technique may serve as a marker for total cell number.

The technique provides a quantitative method for following the growth of any organ. With respect to the brain, the following questions may be raised, even if some cannot be answered at this time: Can normal growth patterns of organs be described in terms of the increase in cell numbers vs. the increase in the size of individual cells? Can alterations in the environment affect normal growth as defined in these terms? What are the mechanisms?

Results of studies of the pattern of DNA increase in different organs in the rat from before birth to 120 days of age were summarized by Dr. Winick. Growth in most organs in the rat continues up to about 100 days, when such growth is measured in terms of increase in weight or protein content of the organ. However, DNA content attains a maximum before growth ceases in all organs.

With respect to the brain, DNA content peaks earliest of all the organs at about 21 days postnatally. The remainder of growth largely reflects an increase in cell size. Thus the early period of growth can be defined as due to an increase in cell number, whereas the later period of growth represents an increase in size of existing cells.

Definition of these two phases of growth permits interpretation of some of the effects of early and late malnutrition. Early malnutrition affects organ growth permanently; malnutrition later in the growth phase will cause an organ to grow improperly, although recovery is possible upon normal feeding. If cells are rapidly dividing, malnutrition impedes the rate of cell division: fewer cells are produced and the change is permanent. Malnutrition during the period when cells are normally enlarging prevents that enlargement: cells will be smaller, but upon refeeding they will resume their normal size by taking up protein.

To understand malnutrition effects on brain, they must be studied at very early developmental stages. Since different parts of the brain undergo different temporal patterns of growth, it can be expected that the effects of malnutrition will vary. The rate of DNA synthesis is most rapid in the cerebellum and stops at about 17 days postnatally in the rat. This rate is slower in the cerebrum and stops at about 21 days. In the brain stem there is little DNA synthesis after the 14th day.

The pattern of development of the hippocampus differs somewhat from other brain regions. In this structure a significant increase in DNA content occurs between the 14th and 17th day. This corresponds to a migration of cells from under the region of the lateral ventricle into the hippocampus, as shown in studies of others.

Malnutrition from birth affects the cerebrum to a moderate degree at about 14 days. The cerebellum is affected quite markedly by 8 days. This confirms the observation that those areas in which cell division occurs most rapidly are those most likely to be affected by severe malnutrition imposed during the time of cell division.

Studies using tritiated thymidine have indicated that malnutrition affects all cell types, provided they are dividing. In the cerebral cortex of the postnatal rat, since no neurons divide, malnutrition does not affect neuron number. On the other hand, malnutrition affects the glia. In the cerebellum, all the cell types which divide postnatally are affected by malnutrition.

These quantitative methods are applicable to studies on the human brain. DNA content increases linearly in the human brain until about birth, then levels off until about 1 year of age when DNA synthesis is completed. Studies of children who died of severe marasmus in Santiago, Chile, revealed a reduced number of cells in the brain, a finding in agreement with observations on rats. However, there are different sequences of events in the human and rat brain. Postnatally, the total DNA content of the cerebrum increases more rapidly than in the cerebellum. All three regions, cerebrum, cerebellum, and brain stem, tend to stop synthesizing DNA about the same time, somewhere around 1 year of age.

In contrast to findings in the rat, a marked and early effect of malnutrition is observed in the cerebrum of the human infant. The basic conclusion, however, is noted, i.e., that severe malnutrition inhibits cell division if cell division is measured by serial analysis of DNA content. In general, a similar conclusion can be drawn by using DNA polymerase activity measurements as a marker of cell division.

Attempts to define further the effects of malnutrition have led to additional studies on RNA metabolism. In work with Rosso and Nelson, Dr. Winick studied RNase activity and RNA and DNA content in normal rat brain from 14 days postconception to 35 days of age. These data were compared to those in animals malnourished during the gestational and lactational periods. RNase content per cell drops initially at birth, followed by a slow increase to 6 days of age, then a period of rapid increase to 14 days, by which time adult levels have been reached. Cell RNA content also increases slowly up to 6 to 8 days and then more rapidly until adult RNA/DNA ratios are reached at 14 to 17 days. When RNase is expressed per mg of RNA, there is a sharp drop at birth to 50% of the previous activity. This lasts 4 days, then increases to previous levels by 10 days of age.

In the malnourished group, RNase per cell is higher up

to 10 days, at which time the rise in RNase in the control brains overtakes the malnourished brains and both values are similar. However, RNase per mg of RNA is persistently higher than normal and there is a smaller increment in the RNA/DNA ratio after the 6th day of age in the malnourished groups.

These data suggest that one mechanism by which malnutrition influences cellular growth may be by affecting the activity of alkaline RNase. Inasmuch as the most significant phases of brain growth occur *in utero,* Dr. Winick, his associates, and others have been concerned that the brain of the undernourished fetus might be damaged by the time of birth. Two types of fetal malnutrition have been studied in animals: maternal protein restriction and uterine artery clamping. The results, at least as far as the fetal brain is concerned, are quite different and suggest the possibility that two types of intrauterine growth failure may occur. When the mother is malnourished from the 4th day of gestation until term, the rate of cell division is curtailed in all fetal organs, including brain. All areas of fetal brain which have been studied are affected by 16 days of gestation. In contrast, uterine artery clamping results in a disproportional effect on the fetal organs. After 6 days of clamping, fetal liver shows a 50% decrease in DNA content, whereas fetal brain shows no effect. In both of these situations, the over-all reduction in body weight of the fetus is the same.

The only cellular data presently available in the human concern placenta. They demonstrate that severe maternal undernutrition will curtail cell division in human placenta. Indirect evidence would also support the contention that the brains of infants who have been exposed to "malnutrition" *in utero* are more sensitive to the effects of postnatal undernutrition. Studies in the area of fetal nutrition therefore become extremely important in the human. The greatest obstacle to developing these studies would appear to be the lack of an adequate "marker" of fetal growth and nutritional status. The use of amniotic fluid as an indicator of fetal genetic makeup has prompted a number of investigators to explore the possibility that changes in the composition of amniotic fluid during development might reflect changes in excretion in fetal metabolites. Hence, if the proper metabolite were found, it might be a marker of growth. The possibilities of using amniotic fluid, nondialyzable hydroxyproline, and amniotic fluid RNase concentration for this purpose will be explored by Dr. Winick's laboratory in future studies.

Discussion of Dr. Winick's presentation focused on the type of malnutrition examined in his studies. He indicated that the prenatal data in animals was produced by putting animals on an isocaloric diet of 5% protein (protein malnutrition). However, since animals on this diet also tend to eat less, the malnutrition represented some caloric as well as protein deprivation. Postnatal restriction was produced by increasing the size of the nursery litter or protein-malnourishing the mother. This reduces the amount of milk, yielding young animals exhibiting both total caloric and protein restriction.

The human cases, who were bottle-fed rather than breast-fed, and almost entirely on a diet of starch and water, underwent a total caloric and protein reduction.

The question also arose concerning the influence of decreasing mothering or environmental deprivation (i.e., sensory or maternal). According to Dr. Winick, some of the studies attempted to control for these possibly disturbing factors. He concluded that the main factor was malnutrition and not environmental alterations.

It was pointed out that there is a fair amount of polyploidy developing in many neurons of the CNS at a critical stage of synaptogenesis. In response to a question whether this polyploidy might be a factor to be considered in the DNA studies, Dr. Winick replied that ploidy is not a concern as long as it is constant. He also discounted the possible role of cell death as a factor in decreasing the rate of DNA synthesis with malnutrition.

# The Limitations of Using a Colchicine-Binding Assay for the Study of Microtubule Protein during Development

E. M. Shooter, J. R. Bamburg, and L. Wilson

As reported by Dr. Shooter and his colleagues, colchicine, an alkaloid produced by *Colchicum autumnale,* has been shown to interrupt cell division (Eigsti and Dustin, 1955), its mechanism of mitotic blockage being due to a specific interaction of the drug with the subunits of microtubules which make up part of the spindle apparatus (Wilson and Friedkin, 1967; Borisy and Taylor, 1967a). Colchicine has also been shown to disrupt microtubules (neurotubules) in nerve fibers (Inoue and Sato, 1967), an event which is followed by retraction of the fiber into the cell body (Daniels, 1968). Using radioactive colchicine, Wilson and Friedkin (1967) showed that the drug was bound specifically to a 105,000 molecular weight protein in grasshopper embryos, and they postulated that this protein was a microtubule subunit. Weisenberg et al. (1968) isolated the colchicine-binding protein from mammalian brain, finding a single component of 120,000 molecular weight. On the basis of circumstantial evidence, they identified it as a subunit protein of microtubules.

An assay method for this colchicine-binding protein arose from the studies on grasshopper embryos by Wilson and Friedkin (1967) and on sea urchin embryos by Borisy and Taylor (1967a). It was later modified by Weisenberg et al. (1968). The procedure, which measures protein-bound colchicine, has been used by many different laboratories to estimate microtubule protein from such diverse sources as mammalian brain (Weisenberg et al., 1968; Redburn and Dahl, 1971; Feit and Barondes, 1970), sea urchin and grasshopper embryos (Wilson and Friedkin, 1967; Borisy and Taylor, 1967a), mouse neuroblastoma cells (Olmsted et al., 1970), and human platelets (Puszkin et al., 1971).

However, in a study of the colchicine-binding activity in chick embryo and brain, Wilson (1970) found a linear response between colchicine binding and protein concentration over a wide range of dilutions and also found that small changes in pH, ionic strength, and temperature greatly affected the rate at which the microtubule protein lost its ability to bind colchicine. The decay rate for the colchicine-binding ability was first order. Changing either the pH or ionic strength of the assay resulted in a different rate of decay ($T_{1/2}$) but had no effect on the initial binding activity. This value, obtained by extrapolation of a decay curve back to zero time, is called the "initial binding capacity (IBC)" and is expressed in terms of dpm of bound $^3$H-colchicine per $\mu$g of protein.

According to Dr. Shooter, who summarized these colchicine studies (with J. R. Bamburg and L. Wilson), in any assay system involving the binding of a radioactive substance to a receptor, it is necessary to have a method for determining binding activity specificity. For colchicine binding, Wilson (1970) showed that, by incubating the assay sample at 0° with colchicine or by adding podophyllotoxin to the assay mixture, most of the colchicine binding could be inhibited. In cases of nonspecific binding of colchicine, little inhibition due to the above conditions was found. It has also been shown that the vinca alkaloids stabilize the colchicine-binding activity of microtubule protein, an effect not seen in the case of nonspecific binding. Therefore, Dr. Shooter noted, in the assay for specific colchicine-binding protein in any tissue, the specificity of the binding must be determined.

In investigations on chick dorsal root ganglia, specificity studies on supernatant from homogenized 12-day-old embryos showed that the colchicine-binding activity responded to 0° incubation and treatment with podophyllotoxin and vincristine sulfate, as did chick brain microtubule protein (Wilson, 1970;

Bamburg et al., 1971). Ganglia (90 to 180) from 7- to 16-day embryos were removed, and, using standard conditions for homogenization, centrifugation, and incubation, decay curves for each age were determined. Protein concentration in the samples was determined by measuring $OD_{210}$ using a value of $\Sigma_{210}^{1.0\%} = 21$. A plot of log dpm per $\mu g$ of protein vs. pre-incubation time was made. The initial binding capacities were determined by extrapolation to zero time, and the half-life of each curve was measured. Large changes in both the half-life (Fig. 4) and IBC (Fig. 5) were observed. Because the changes in $T_{1/2}$ were decreasing with age and IBC was increasing, the curves all came close to crossing at the 2-hour point of incubation. A fixed time colchicine-binding assay done at this time would have shown virtually no change in the amount of colchicine-binding protein (Fig. 5). To determine whether the changes in amount of colchicine-binding protein were real, extracts from ganglia that had been saved were reduced, carboxymethylated, and run, along with purified reduced and carboxymethylated microtubule protein, on 8 M urea acrylamide gels using a tris-glycinate buffer system. Staining the gel

**Figure 4.** The variation of colchicine binding half-life with development in homogenized embryonic chick ganglia. (Figures 4, 5, and 6 are preliminary versions of data given in Bamburg, J. R., Shooter, E. M., and Wilson, L. 1973. Assay of microtubule protein in embryonic chick dorsal root ganglia. Neurobiology in press.)

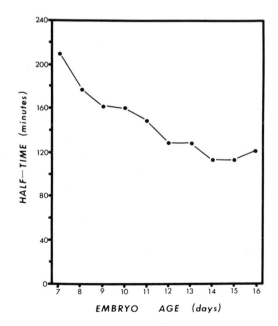

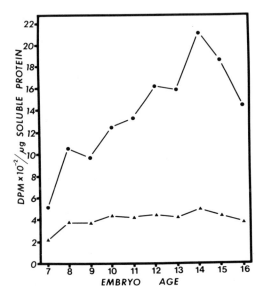

**Figure 5.** Comparison of time-decay (●) and single point (▲) colchicine-binding activity in supernatants of homogenized ganglia. The *bottom curve* is the data obtained by use of the first colchicine-binding point of each decay assay (2 hours of incubation).

with acid-fast green gave a linear response for the microtubule protein when area of the peak of a scanned gel was plotted against protein concentration. Concentrations of microtubule protein in the ganglia homogenates were determined (Fig. 6) and found to correspond to the changes seen in IBC and not to the fixed time colchicine-binding assay results. Therefore, Dr. Shooter noted, in any system under study, where the half-life of the colchicine-binding ability of the protein may be changing, microtubule protein must be measured by using IBC and not fixed time assays.

In attempting to accumulate statistically accurate changes in developing ganglia, a large variation of IBC's within ganglia of the same age was found. When ganglia were pooled, homogenized, then divided into fractions for individual curves, a much smaller amount of variation was found. The problem in variability, therefore, resided either in the ganglia themselves or in the homogenization step. Sonication was thus tried to solubilize the ganglial proteins. Sonicated ganglia from embryos of the same age gave very reproducible decay curves, but very little, if any, difference could be noted on ganglia from 8 to 12 days of development. The changes seen originally must, therefore, have been artifacts of the homogenization procedure.

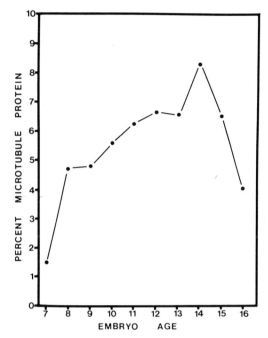

**Figure 6.** Percentage of microtubule protein, determined by polyacrylamide gel electrophoresis, in supernatant fractions of homogenized ganglia from different age chick embryos.

## EXPERIMENTS ON CHICK EMBRYO BRAIN

To evaluate the use of initial binding capacities for determining microtubule protein in developing tissue, embryonic and postembryonic chick brain was used in place of ganglia because of its size and ease of extraction from the embryo. Brains were disrupted by sonication and assayed for colchicine-binding activity, as was described for ganglia, except that a lower specific activity $^3$H-colchicine was used.

Variation within samples of brains of the same age was evident, and significant results were obtained only by determining four to eight decay curves for each age of brain. Variation seemed to be greater on samples of the same age done on different days than if they were done together on the same day. Statistical analysis of the data was done using Student's t test at a 95% confidence level. The initial binding capacities were determined by a computer using the method of least squares and extrapolation to zero time.

The earliest embryos in which brains could be easily removed were 5 days old, and an increasing amount of binding activity was found in brain from this age up to 13 days of

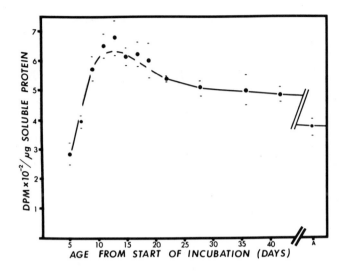

**Figure 7.** Changes in initial binding capacity in supernatant fractions of sonicated chick brain of different ages. (Figures 7 and 9 are from data given in Bamburg, J. R., Shooter, E. M., and Wilson, L., 1973. Developmental changes in microtubule protein of chick brain. Biochemistry (Washington) in press.)

development (Fig. 7). Following this period there was a gradual decline in the IBC up to adulthood (6 months old). The decline seen in the IBC at embryo ages older than 13 days seemed to be coupled with a change in the ratio of soluble to particulate protein. An assay of brain sonicates for total and soluble protein (after centrifugation) showed a steady decline in the amount of soluble protein (Fig. 8). Therefore, the possibility remained that much of the colchicine-binding activity was being lost in the particulate protein fraction.

When specificity tests were run on soluble and particulate fractions of homogenized brain, the colchicine-binding activity in both responded like the purified microtubule protein (MTP).

The amount of colchicine-binding protein actually in the particulate fraction was measured by doing the binding assay on the whole sonicate of different aged brains and centrifuging down the particulate binding material. After several washes, the particulate protein was counted. From limited data now available, it appears that very little particulate binding occurs in embryo brains younger than 13 days. The total dpm

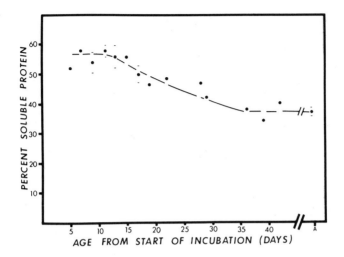

**Figure 8.** Variation of total and soluble protein in supernatant fractions of sonicated chick brain of different ages.

in both soluble and particulate does not decline in brains older than 13 days when expressed in terms of total dpm per $\mu$g of soluble protein. To Dr. Shooter this suggests that the particulate binding may be due to entrapped MTP which was not solubilized on the first sonication. Resonication of these samples released an additional 20% of the trapped colchicine-binding activity. Since myelinization of neuronal fibers starts at about 13 days of embryonic development in the chick embryo, it is not surprising to find an increase of entrapped MTP at this stage. If one expressed the IBC in terms of total protein (soluble and particulate) in the brain, then there is definitely a decline in total dpm per $\mu$g of total protein following 13 days of embryonic development in chick brain.

In summary, there is an increase in the amount of microtubule protein relative to other proteins (both soluble and particulate) up to 13 days of development. Following this period, the amount of MTP stays about constant in proportion to the soluble protein of the brain but decreases when compared to total protein, probably because of myelin formation and other particulate membrane proteins.

A statistically significant difference (95% confidence level) in half-life also was found for the colchicine-binding activity in

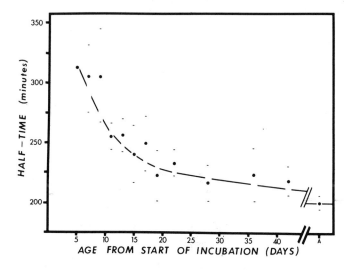

**Figure 9.** Changes in colchicine binding half-life in supernatant fractions of sonicated chick brain of different ages.

brains of different ages. The younger embryos had a higher $T_{1/2}$ (Fig. 9) (just as was seen in ganglia) and gradually decreased until by 18 days of embryonic development the $T_{1/2}$ changed little. In Dr. Shooter's opinion, changes in $T_{1/2}$ would certainly make the single point colchicine-binding assays less accurate in measuring changes in microtubule protein during development than if decay curves were used to obtain the initial binding capacities.

# Methodological Problems in Studying the Developing Brain

**N. Radin**

To aid in defining critical areas for research in mental retardation, Dr. Radin proposed several avenues in which new or greater activity is needed. He views them as potential contractual projects for NIH to develop.

**1.** Improved methods are needed for homogenizing brains and preparing subcellular fractions. Few people seem to have taken advantage of the publications describing tissue homogenizers which are rigidly mounted, have controlled, reproducible choices of speed, and use continuous flow. A specific clearance between rotating pestle and cooled jacket should be offered, instead of the vague clearances in most current homogenizers. No commercial homogenizer of this sort is available, yet it is known from several published studies and many private ones over a long period of time that subcellular distributions vary with the individual, the day, and the laboratory. This trivial mechanical problem should be brought under control.

Subcellular fractionation methods have made great progress, but many membranes appear in several overlapping fractions and a considerable portion of each brain homogenate ends up as ill defined vesicles and fragments. The invention of the zonal centrifuge looked like a promising addition to the field, but surprisingly few techniques have come from it. One difficulty is that each experiment consumes a great deal of gradient medium and anything more expensive than sucrose is very expensive. Perhaps the centrifuge manufacturers should offer a small zonal rotor that will permit research scientists to try different gradient systems more economically and to use less tissue per run.

Another approach that has not lived up to its promise yet, according to Dr. Radin, is the complexing of membranes with specific compounds. This method has proved quite successful in the isolation of lysosomes following the injection into animals of Triton WR-1339. Lysosomes take up part of the Triton, change their density, and become separable by centrifugation. This method must be adaptable to other membranous particles, perhaps by mixing them in specific antibodies coupled to dense molecules.

2. For analyzing brain lipids, improved micromethods are needed, comparable to gas chromatography and amino acid chromatography. The lipid neurochemists lag far behind the gas and ion exchange chromatographers in terms of speed, sensitivity, automation, and detail of data. Because the former are handicapped by the high molecular weight of most lipids, gas chromatography is probably out of the question. Owing to a lack of ionized groups (except for a few lipids) ion exchange chromatography is also unfeasible. No automated method, such as the flame ionization detector or the ninhydrin reaction, is yet available for measuring microscopic amounts of every type of lipid.

Perhaps the new high pressure liquid chromatographic systems being offered commercially can be used advantageously. These use new packing materials, of very low particle size, requiring the use of hundreds of pounds of pressure to drive solvents through the columns. Very high resolving power is achieved by using long columns; these are practical because of the powerful pumps. Industrial laboratories are getting excellent results with this approach. Dr. Radin believes that the more conservative biochemists should try it as well. He likened the current situation to the early days of gas chromatography, when the petroleum companies were making intense use of the technique while the biochemists waited for them to work out the mechanical problems.

In Dr. Radin's view, the new super-sensitive column monitors that come with these systems look very promising for compounds which absorb in the ultraviolet region. Reasonable peaks are obtained with *only* 5 mg of nucleosides when the instrument is set at 0.01 OD full scale. Such a system should be relatively simple to use with many compounds of importance to the brain, such as the catecholamines. As with gas chromatography, in which conversion of nonvolatile compounds by silylation has worked wonders, it should be possible to render many substances detectable by derivation with an aromatic reagent, such as benzoyl chloride. In this way the system could probably be adapted to analysis of amino acids, $\gamma$-aminobutyric acid, hydroxy compounds, histamine, and the new behavioral peptides.

If liquid chromatographic systems of this type could be developed for brain lipids and assorted compounds, Dr. Radin believes it would be possible to carry out detailed examination of microscopically small brain biopsy samples. The changes seen in lipidoses could be elucidated in great depth. Blood analysis would become feasible for children, from whom only small volumes are available. Using animal brains, one could analyze in detail each type of subcellular particle and brain region and evaluate attempts at intervening in the process of brain maturation.

**3.** One field which needs more trials is the experimental intervention in the maturation process. There have been publications on some of the effects of thyroidectomy and thyroid replacement, of growth hormone supplementation, and of psychoactive drugs. Food deprivation is a currently popular interventional tool. To Dr. Radin, this approach must owe its attractiveness to an ethical empathy rather than to its biochemical promise, for he views it as the least specific chemical technique imaginable. Perhaps contractors should study the effects on maturation of addicting drugs, alcohol, home remedies, high levels of vitamin C, pollutants, and the toxins resulting from overpopulation and overtechnology. A host of assays are needed: behavioral, chemical, electrophysiological, and microscopic. Each neurochemical assay should be chromatographic, to get as much data as possible from each animal. Dr. Radin observed that this is bound to be called "mindless research," without a rationale, which may lead to no findings or to uninterpretable findings. However, he believes that exciting leads could very well come from such experiments. The rationale will take care of itself after the finding is made. Putting it differently, the researcher is a hero *after* he discovers that aspirin cures headaches.

**4.** Another neglected field, in Dr. Radin's view, is the development of inhibitors for specific enzymes in the brain. Spectacular advances have come from the development of inhibitors for the enzymes which metabolize the psychoactive amines, such as monoamine oxidase and cholinesterase. A number of additional brain-specific compounds cannot now be manipulated by synthetic compounds. Until this sort of specific manipulation can be carried out, progress in understanding the function of these compounds will be slow and it may be difficult to help children who have a metabolic disorder of one of these compounds.

Dr. Radin believes that many neurochemists are ready for this stage in research. Assay systems for some of the enzymes have been developed; it would be a simple matter to synthesize and test compounds similar to the substrates. The pharmaceutical companies cannot be looked to for potentially suitable compounds because there is no rationale yet in controlling any particular enzyme a neurochemist might choose to study. Thus each researcher must hire one of the many available organic chemists with a biological bent and interest him in the subject.

**5.** The same sort of synthetic organic chemistry is called for in the investigation of cell surface interactions. This is a new, exciting field, but it is moving slowly. It seems highly likely to Dr. Radin that the polysaccharide regions of glycoproteins or glycolipids are actively concerned with the migration, aggregation, and other contact phenomena of cells. These are activities of quintessential importance in the developing brain, in which axons aim themselves at specific neurons and cells migrate in fantastic choreography. Artificial analogues of polysaccharides are needed which will block these interactions to allow identification of specific stages in brain development in specific regions. Perhaps such compounds would allow disaggregation of specific cells and yield the pure, isolated cells for detailed study.

**6.** There is need for a preparation center, like the two or so now set up for large scale protein isolations. Semipilot works are needed where scientists can come to prepare adequate amounts of substrates, radioactive materials, and potential enzyme inhibitors. A permanent staff should guide the investigator in scaling up his procedure, and a portion of the product should be retained by the center for later sale or processing.

The prices of commercially available lipids, for example, are fantastically high. Large scale procedures must be developed for isolating or synthesizing compounds of special interest in research with the developing brain. Since there is no obvious pharmacological significance to this, small scale commercial labs must be relied upon for the time being.

7. Another need cited by Dr. Radin is for the development of detergents that are readily degraded by a purified enzyme. Apparently membranous enzymes, which account for many of the most interesting reactions in the brain, cannot be solubilized and purified unless a detergent is added to the membrane. Tritons and Tweens have been popular, but these are difficult to remove from the enzyme. If one tries to carry out a column purification using the detergent in the eluting liquid, it is difficult to concentrate the enzyme without carrying along excessive amounts of detergent. It should be possible to devise a detergent which will extract enzymes without hurting them and can be hydrolyzed by some commercially available hydrolytic enzyme. Of course, the products of hydrolysis should be easily removed, say by extraction with hexane or dialysis. Lysolecithin might be appropriate, although at present it is exorbitantly expensive. Tweens are esters, in part, and it should be possible to degrade them with a purified lipase.

8. Another project is needed to solve the many problems of literature awareness and bibliography maintenance. Dr. Radin suggested several approaches, of varying complexity and expense. A simple one consists in using the annual reports sent by grantees to the National Institute of Child Health and Human Development, the National Institute of Neurological Diseases and Stroke, and the National Institute of Mental Health. These reports list the publications by each grantee for the past year. If such lists could be compiled and sent out to workers in the field, researchers could more readily keep track of current work and read articles that might otherwise be missed. The selectivity of the list would act to make it particularly useful. It could be issued monthly for maximal timeliness.

In a somewhat more sophisticated approach, the bibliography could be selective for each individual worker. Each investigator in the field of mental retardation would send NIH his list of key words. If any title contained one of those words, the bibliographic reference would be printed out by the NIH computer and the assembled list mailed every month to each individual. A similar search could be made for key names, so that the work of individual colleagues could be followed. This type of alertness service would probably not be too expensive. In contrast to the very comprehensive commercially operated alerting services, this one would be quite restricted and the cost of searching the magnetically stored information would be correspondingly small.

**9.** Dr. Radin also recommended, only somewhat tongue-in-cheek, the formation of a special consumer-oriented task force (perhaps under NIH sponsorship) to monitor publications from brain research laboratories. Similar monitoring for manufacturers of chemicals and equipment was also suggested.

# SESSION III.
# MORPHOPHYSIO-LOGICAL STUDIES OF BRAIN MATURATION

# Approaches: Advantages and Limitations

**D. P. Purpura**

Morphophysiological approaches to the study of brain maturation have generally been based on the premise that examining
the sequential elaboration of neuronal and synaptic subsystems
and their respective electrophysiological properties will yield
important structure-function correlations otherwise obscured
by the overwhelming complexity of the mature brain (Purpura, 1961). According to Dr. Purpura, this premise implies
two assumptions: 1) that the morphogenesis of neurons and
their synaptic relations can be specified with a fair degree of
precision; and 2) that alterations in electrophysiological events
can be related to specific features of the morphogenetic process.

For the most part, studies which seek to answer questions
about the manner in which morphogenetic changes are
reflected in electrophysiological events have rarely dealt with
behavioral concomitants of normal development, if one ex-
cludes from consideration the analysis of simple reflex activities. On the other hand, alterations in behavioral development
have been sought in response to a wide variety of hormonal,
traumatic, and environmental perturbations. Attempts have
been made to correlate end-stage effects with gross morphological and/or physiological parameters of brain maturation.
The lack of adequate criteria for assessing quantitative as well
as qualitative aspects of normal brain maturation in morphophysiological terms has not at all dampened the enthusiasm for identifying abnormalities of development. Dr.
Purpura identified a number of key questions which are likely
to specify important research strategies for morphophysiological studies.

First and foremost are questions pertaining to processes which control and program the elaboration of *dendrites* of neurons, particularly in cortical structures, which exhibit the most profound maturational changes in the postnatal period in altricial mammals. An obvious question is, "Why dendrites?" One might answer that the phylogenesis of neurons is expressed in a progressive elaboration of the dendritic trees as major synaptic receptor surfaces of neurons. For the typical pyramidal neurons of mammalian cerebral cortex, more than 95% of the available surface for synaptic inputs is provided by dendrites. However, not all this surface is covered with synapses. Remarkably enough, probably only 10 to 15% of the entire soma-dendritic surface of cortical pyramidal neurons is occupied by synapses, as defined by the usual electron micro scopic criteria. This figure is similar for the variety of neurons with axons ramifying in cortex which for convenience may be called "interneurons."

According to Dr. Purpura, assessment of the ontogenetic changes in neuronal morphology has been best studied with the Golgi technique or one of its variants (Fig. 10). In general, the Golgi method stains virtually the entire cell body and dendritic tree of 1 to 5% of neurons. Axonal ramifications are variably stained. Several mysteries surround the use of this method. The precise chemical reaction that leads to the lipo-protein-chrome-silver or mercury precipitate inside the chosen few neurons is not known. Similarly, the factors that determine which neurons will be stained are unknown, although functional activities have been suggested as well as rejected. Finally, it is remarkable that staining of adjacent structures is avoided, as Ramon-Moliner (1970) has emphasized. To Dr. Purpura, this last factor renders the Golgi method suspect for the estimation of synaptic contacts, although the identification of dendritic spines as synaptic contact sites has some redeeming value in this respect. Dr. Purpura also pointed out that a number of investigators have used Golgi preparations in statistical studies of dendritic branching patterns. With these approaches it has been possible to transform the Golgi method from a staining technique to a valuable experimental method and to formulate certain relations from data obtained by measuring morphological details such as the size relations between cell body and nucleus, the branching pattern of the dendritic

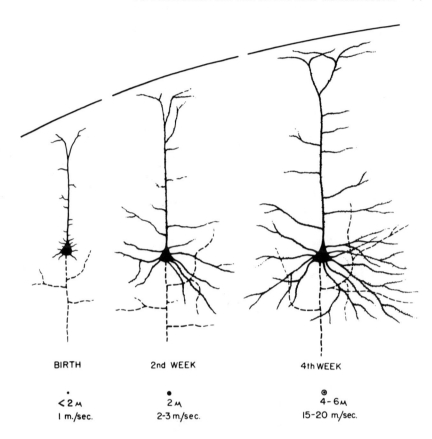

BIRTH     2nd WEEK     4th WEEK

<2 м     2 м     4- 6 м
I m./sec.     2-3 m./sec.     15-20 m./sec.

**Figure 10.** General characteristics of neocortical pyramidal neurons in the kitten at birth, 2 weeks, and 4 weeks postnatally. Relative diameter of axons and conduction velocities of largest fibers in medullary pyramidal tract are indicated below each cell for the different ages. Axons and axon collaterals are shown as *dashed lines.* In the newborn kitten, pyramidal neurons have well developed apical dendrites, and many have rudimentary basilar dendritic systems. Axon collaterals are poorly developed, and dendrites are devoid of typical spines. During the 2 postnatal week basilar dendrites grow extensively, and apical dendrites increase in length and contain more tangential branches. Spines appear on dendrites at this stage, and axon collateral growth is prominent. In the 1-month-old kitten, neocortical pyramidal neurons have attained adult characteristics. Myelination of the largest corticospinal axons is completed by the 4th or 5th month. (Modified from Purpura et al., 1965.)

trees and the axonal network. To the late Dr. Sholl goes the credit for first attempts at defining the functional relationship between the number of intersections of dendrites per unit area and the distance from the center of the cell body, i.e., the connective field of the neuron. The basic method has been elaborated and modified by other workers and applied to normal and abnormal cortical neuronal developmental processes (Valverde, 1970).

In recent years the question of evaluating the contribution of dendritic branching patterns to the functional activity of neurons has become important. Dr. Purpura observed that as a check on the geometrical properties of dendritic branching patterns revealed in Golgi preparations, the introduction of vital staining of neurons with intracellular injection of fluorescent dyes such as procion yellow is refreshing to note. This method has permitted direct calculations of soma-dendritic conductances and other parameters of dendritic characteristics in cells examined electrophysiologically. The technique has yet to be applied to immature mammalian neurons where stable intracellular recording and dye injection are difficult at best.

The postnatal development of dendrites of cortical neurons has been examined in a number of species including man (Purpura and Schade, 1964). Molliver and Van der Loos (1970) have summarized the two basic principles of cortical maturation derived from studies dating back to Vignal and Cajal as follows. Deep cells mature earlier than superficial cells, and apical dendritic growth precedes the growth of basal dendrites. There can be no question that superficial pyramidal neurons have well developed apical dendrites prior to the appearance of their basilar dendrites (Noback and Purpura, 1961). Electron microscopy (EM) has indicated that such superficial apical dendrites are among the earliest sites for synaptic contacts. The application of EM to the study of immature cerebral cortex reported originally by Voeller, Pappas, and Purpura (1963) provided the first morphological evidence of well developed synapses on cortical dendrites in the immediate neonatal period. Since that time it has been proposed as a principle of synaptogenesis that axodendritic synapses are the first interneuronal interrelations established in the mammalian cerebral cortex (Purpura, 1968). Since the publication of this

EM study, additional methods including the phospho-tungstic acid (PTA) staining of synapses in combination with quantitative electron microscopy have been developed by Aghajanian and Bloom (1967). Quantitative EM methods have also begun to answer the important question of *where the first synapses are located in the immature cortex.* A related issue concerns how one evaluates the significance of variable morphological features of neuronal appositions as criteria for defining immature synapses. In Dr. Purpura's view, the importance of this methodological approach cannot be overemphasized.

Synaptogenesis in the mammalian cerebral cortex is characterized by overlapping temporal sequences of synapse formation involving first dendrites, then cell bodies, and the rapid proliferation of axodendritic synapses related to spines. The rarity of axosomatic synapses in neocortex and hippocampus (Schwartz, Pappas, and Purpura, 1968) of newborn kittens is noteworthy. The reason for this is not known, however, and remains a problem of no little importance. Much more must be learned concerning the time course of synaptogenesis and why the cell bodies of some neurons, such as those in the raphé nuclei or pontine reticular formation, are 50 to 80% covered by synaptic profiles whereas others, such as in the caudate nucleus, exhibit rare axosomatic synapses even in adult animals. Apart from these questions, the answers to which will require extensive serial thin sectioning, there is the problem of defining the functional significance of different types of developing synapses, i.e., Type I and Type II, and all the varieties between these two extremes of the synaptic spectrum. Quantitative evaluation of the number, shape, and size of synaptic vesicles has been attempted as well as evaluation of the size and density of axonal terminals and the relationship of vesicle population to specialized components of the presynaptic membrane. Additional parametric data for ontogenetic studies can be obtained by examining the extent of specialized membrane apposition at developing synapses. Many of these analyses require enormous expenditures of time and effort. However, more attention will undoubtedly be paid in the future to the development of relatively simple computer interfacing equipment which, when linked to flying-spot scanning optics, may permit rapid surveys of PTA-stained synaptic regions, vesicle morphology, and other features.

Dr. Purpura injected a word of caution lest it be thought that the use of profile recognition techniques involving computer scanning methods are right around the corner for the neuromorphologist. Such was the belief nearly a decade ago, but experience has dampened the enthusiasm of even the most enterprising. For the present Dr. Purpura believes there is no substitute for well trained eyeballs fitted to the head bone of an imaginative neurobiologist capable of asking the right questions, at the right time, when looking at optimally prepared material.

Turning to the question of dendritic spines, Dr. Purpura noted that it has certainly occupied the attention of more neurobiologists in recent years than seems justified simply on the basis of physiological significance, which is as yet completely unknown. In adult animals, experimental degeneration techniques combined with EM have recently suggested that, at least in primary projection areas of cortex, dendritic spines are the sites of contact for a large proportion of thalamocortical, interhemispheric, and intrahemispheric afferents (Jones and Powell, 1970). Changes in spine shape, number, and distribution have been observed in a variety of experimental situations including sensory deprivation (Valverde, 1970) and local metabolic and traumatic alterations which are associated with the appearance of chronic epileptogenic activities (Westrum et al., 1964). In this context, Dr. Purpura noted with interest that Valverde and Ruiz-Marcos (1969) have defined a mathematical model for estimating the distribution of spines along the apical dendrites.

The spine question was considered in some detail by Dr. Purpura not only to emphasize the importance of developing quantitative methods for assessing dendritic spines but to point out some questions which remain unanswered. For example, does a change in spine number or distribution as revealed in Golgi material reflect a true change in spine population or a failure to impregnate spines following some particular intervention? What about the question of assessing changes in synaptic organization in immature cortex prior to the period of spine proliferation? And finally, what are spines for?

Dr. Purpura and his associates have been particularly interested in these questions in view of physiological data indicating that primary projection activity is clearly detectable in the neocortex of newborn altricial mammals (before spine elaboration). Primary evoked potentials have electrographic characteristics which are attributable to superficial axodendritic postsynaptic events. If such is indeed the case, then the burden of the proof rests with Dr. Purpura's group to demonstrate superficially distributing primary afferents in immature cortex. To do so, experimental degeneration techniques of light and electron microscopy must be applied to the study of the developing brain. Studies in this direction in Dr. Purpura's laboratory constitute the first attempts to utilize the Fink-Heimer technique in conjunction with EM observations following lesions of thalamocortical and other projection systems in the young kitten. The problems in this research strategy are numerous since attempts to reveal degeneration in cortex with silver impregnation techniques are difficult at best in mature animals and the question of evaluating the response of immature axons and axon terminals to degeneration are formidable indeed. These methods obviously require the hottest pursuit in immature animals. In Dr. Purpura's opinion, more must be known concerning the factors influencing dendritic growth, distribution, and orientation, as well as the pattern of normal and abnormal synaptogenesis (including the mode of engagement of cortical neurons by developing afferent projection and intracortical pathways). Until then, little can be said about the significance of more molar features of brain maturation in the postnatal period such as brain weight, gray/white coefficients, and cell body and neuropil density. Many factors will undoubtedly be found which influence the pattern of dendritic growth which in itself is a major determinant of intracortical microcircuitry.

Apart from the morphological problems concerning parameters of brain maturation, several key questions have arisen in studies of the developmental physiology of the mammalian brain. There are first questions which are physiological analogues of morphological inquiries, such as: What are the properties of immature neurons and synapses? What is the relationship between myelination and conduction velocity in different subsystems of axonal pathways? How are morphogenetic alterations in cortical neuronal organizations reflected in evoked potential changes? How do patterns of discharges in immature neurons change with development, and what does this signify? A second category of questions encompasses more global problems linking electrophysiological and behavioral considerations, for example, the question of evaluating the ontogenesis of sleep-wakefulness activities and their relationship to the maturation of different brain stem organizations.

The first class of questions has been approached largely by the use of macro- as well as microphysiological techniques for unit and intracellular recording. For obvious reasons there have been relatively few reports of successful intracellular recordings in immature cortical neurons (Fig. 11). The method has, however, disclosed the low level excitability and lack of high frequency repetitive responsiveness of immature neurons in the very early postnatal period. Intracellular recording has also established that excitatory and inhibitory synaptic activities in cortex do not develop equipotently in the immediate postnatal period.

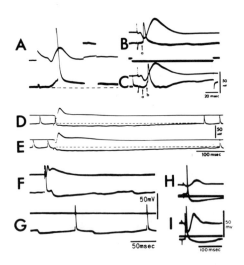

**Figure 11.** Examples of spike potentials and synaptic activities intracellularly recorded from neocortical and hippocampal neurons in the neonatal and young kitten. *A:* Prolonged EPSP (80 to 100 msec) evoked by ventrolateral thalamic stimulation in a sensorimotor cortex neuron from a 6-day-old kitten. In this and other dual channel recordings, the upper channel records indicate cortical surface activity, negativity upwards. Weak stimulation elicits an 18- to 20-msec latency EPSP with a slow rise time and prolonged declining phase.

does the relatively simple, immature synapse pattern develop into the complex, mature pattern?). Perhaps correlations can be established between structurally definable synapse layers and the nature of evoked responses in various stages of development. These researchers hope to arrive at *physiologically determinable* stages of synapse development ("circuitry age"). Norms may be defined, then applied in evaluating degree of maturity in control and experimental conditions (animals) and, later, in health and disease (human).

# Electrophysiological Approaches to Developmental Studies

M. Bennett

In discussing the function of dendritic spines and the significance of junctions coupling embryonic cells, Dr. Bennett saw little electrophysiological significance in a dendritic spine of the ordinary sort. However, he noted that possible function has been proposed in a preliminary form by Llinás and Hillman (1969). They suggested that the neck of a dendritic spine provides a series resistance which causes the spine to act as a constant current source, thereby leading to more linear summation of inputs.

According to their argument, measurements of spines on Purkinje cells allowed a calculated "neck" resistance of about 10 M$\Omega$ (0.2 $\mu$ diameter, 0.5 $\mu$ length, 60 $\Omega$ cm core resistivity). Further assuming a "head" of 2 $\mu$ diameter and surface resistivity of 1000 $\Omega$ cm$^2$, one calculates a head surface resistance of 10$^{10}$ $\Omega$. The minimum size of a postsynaptic potential (PSP) at the synapse on the spine may be taken as one quantum or vesicle which at the neuromuscular junction introduces a shunt resistance of about 17 M$\Omega$ (Gage and Armstrong, 1968).

The equivalent circuits of a single spine and dendrite to which it is attached are diagrammed in Fig. 12$A$. An isopotential region of dendrite is considered with few enough spines so that the resistance of all the spines in parallel, $(r_{surf} + r_{neck})/n$, is large compared to the input resistance. This allows a fair number of spines as indicated from the computed input resistance for very long 2-$\mu$ and 10-$\mu$ diameter dendrites (assuming 1000 $\Omega$ cm$^2$ membrane resistivity). The resistance $r_{active}$ represents the synaptic membrane on the spine during its activity. Since $r_{surf}$ is also very large compared to the maximum value of

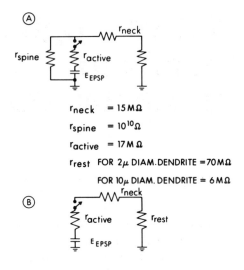

Figure 12

$r_{active}$ (which would be at most that for one quantum of trans-mitter), $r_{surf}$ can be omitted. Several points become obvious from inspection of the new simplified circuit (Fig. 12B). If one lets $r_a = r_{active} + r_{neck}$, the circuit is identical to that for a synapse on an ordinary isopotential cell except that the internal resistance of the synaptic generator is larger. Hence, summation of more parallel inputs (each on a separate spine) is required to give the same depolarization in the axis of the dendrite than if the inputs were on the dendrite shaft. Llinás and Hillman pointed out that, because in the assumed circuit the relation between potential and synaptic conductance (or number of inputs active) is more linear for small depolarizations, the same number of spine inputs produces a smaller voltage and gives a more linear summation. However, summation of more parallel spine inputs is required to give the same depolarization that inputs on the shaft would produce. In Dr. Bennett's opinion, it seems more meaningful to consider the relation between po-tential and fraction of inputs required to give the same final dendritic depolarization in the two cases. This relation is iden-tical whether or not the inputs are on spines. For example, if 16 spinal inputs and 8 shaft inputs are required to give the same depolarization, then 4, 8, and 12 inputs in the first case give the same potentials as 2, 4, and 6 inputs in the second case. The input-output relations have the same shape.

The neck resistance of a spine does allow a somewhat smaller quantum size (by a factor of about two assuming that the excitatory postsynaptic potential (EPSP) quantum size is the same as that at the neuromuscular junction). However, if smaller quanta were desirable, the animal could have evolved them in at least two other ways: by reducing the amount of transmitter per vesicle or by reducing the postsynaptic sensitivity to the transmitter.

Dr. Bennett noted that even the largest value of $r_{active}$, that for a single neuromuscular quantum, is significant in terms of the calculated dendritic input resistance, $r_{rest}$. Thus, the minimum size EPSP may be a substantial depolarization. One rather remotely possible function of spines can be derived from this consideration. If $r_{active}$ involves many quanta, variability becomes less, but the minimum for $r_a$ is still $r_{neck}$. Thus a relatively small but less variable PSP might be obtained. Dr. Bennett has observed that other and more efficient mechanisms of reducing PSP variability below that of a Poisson distribution are conceivable (Auerbach and Bennett, 1969). If $r_{spine}$ is quite small (much smaller than $r_{neck}$), the circuit can give more linear summation of inputs than with an isopotential cell. The situation becomes comparable to summation in a soma of inputs arising far out on different dendrites. This arrangement greatly hinders inversion of PSPs by applied currents; thus, to Dr. Bennett it does not seem relevant, at least to climbing fiber PSPs in the Purkinje cell (see Llinás and Hillman, 1969).

As another possibility, one might consider the role of spines in ionic concentration changes within the spine during a response. Although ionic movements during a miniature PSP could be a significant fraction of the ions in a spine (something like a 10 mM change), the rate of diffusion out of the spine would be rapid compared to the duration of a response.

Dr. Bennett believes that there is no obvious electrophysiological function of spines. (This statement does not apply to the "giant" spine on fish spinal motoneurons (Diamond and Yasargil, 1969) which is large and equivalent to a dendrite.) One could make ontogenetic arguments of various kinds, but to Dr. Bennett the desirability of doing so with present data is questionable.

Turning to some experiments that had arisen earlier in the symposium, Dr. Bennett observed that there are many experiments which, although feasible, may not give interesting results. One may do extensive counting and obtain highly significant results (statistically) and might even be very clever in the methodology applied, yet learning nothing of true scientific significance. Reliable data, while necessary for the best science, are not sufficient. The experiment must be designed to give a meaningful answer, and the meaning of meaning is not always easy to arrive at.

An illustration of experimental feasibility and significance was taken from Dr. Bennett's work on electrical coupling in embryos. In an attempt to discover how cells communicate with each other in development, Dr. Bennett and a number of other workers have put microelectrodes in embryonic cells and measured electrotonic coupling between cells (Bennett and Trinkaus, 1970). Is this coupling meaningful?

The observations mean that small ions go back and forth between cells. One can, in principle, describe the developmental changes in electrical coupling, although there are very few points in the developmental series available. When the cells are large enough for the electrophysiologist to study them easily, they are coupled. However, they go on being coupled until they are very small, and the experiments become very difficult. Thus, there are few data correlating degree of coupling with developmental stage. Are messages passing between coupled cells which are significant to development? The electrical measurements show that some small ions can go back and forth between them. Permeability measurements show molecules of molecular weight of at least 500 cross junctions in adult tissue (Payton et al., 1969), but the smaller molecule fluorescein (m.w. 332) fails to cross junctions between early embryonic cells (Bennett and Spira, 1971). An attempt is being made to find the message by determining the size of the filter through which the message passes. To Dr. Bennett, while that is not a very direct approach to finding the message, it is feasible. One could infer from the few available permeability data that, if the electrical junctions mediate any molecular communication between the cells at this stage, a molecule smaller than fluorescein is involved. Dr. Bennett believes that this possibility is not absurd, because there are *in vitro* demonstrations that the course of tissue differentiation can be markedly affected by changes in concentrations of small ions (Barth and Barth, 1969; Macklin and Burnett, 1966). Small ions could pass between these cells by way of the electrotonic junctions and thereby influence differentiation.

He sees a permissive case for communication in differentiation by way of these junctions. More information is required concerning when cells are coupled and when they decouple electrically and whether ions actually pass between cells. When cells become small, as they do when differentiating, it may be necessary to use morphological instead of physiological identification of the junctions that couple cells.

To "raise a little uncertainty," Dr. Bennett mentioned the possibility of communication between embryonic cells across extracellular space as well as by way of junctions. Chemical transmission, as at synapses, is another way in which cells communicate; studies of coupling have not revealed whether embryonic cells communicate in that way.

Dr. Bennett made some general proposals concerning the directions in which morphological techniques might advance. A toxin is available which binds to peripheral acetylcholine (ACh) channels (bungarotoxin) very nearly irreversibly (Changeaux et al., 1970; Miledi et al., 1971). Use of this toxin seems to be leading to isolation of the ACh receptor, and use of other toxins for isolation of other channels is at least plausible. If one makes labelled antibodies to the toxins or in some other way makes the toxin molecules identifiable at the EM level, one can begin to think of counting different kinds of channels in different regions of the cells. While perhaps far off, a technique of this sort may be the only one that will allow study of dendrites, because electrodes and amplifiers are unlikely to improve appreciably.

A great deal of electrophysiology involves tracing of pathways, and contributions of conventional morphological studies are still required. To Dr. Bennett it would not be unreasonable to propose mapping by computerized techniques as currently employed in the laboratories of Brenner and Levinthal. These groups are working on small animals at the EM level ($30\text{-}\mu$ diameter ganglia at perhaps 50 Å resolution). Scaling everything up by a factor of 100 should be feasible and could give very important information. Sampling at the EM level, particularly if kinds of synaptic and membrane function can be identified morphologically, might be adequate to give a satisfactory working diagram of, at the very least, small parts of the nervous system. To know the connectivity of the nervous system is a necessary preliminary to understanding it.

# Studies
# in Neuropsychology

**H. Vaughan**

The electrical activity of the intact functioning human brain represents a unique linkage between psychological processes and the underlying neuromechanisms. According to Dr. Vaughan, in theory, recordings of neuroelectric data can provide a moment-by-moment indication of the neural activities which give rise to subjective experience and lead to the emission of externally observable behavior. It is evident, however, that even direct cerebral recordings of gross extracellular potentials or interneural activity in the behaving organism provide but an incomplete and biased picture of the dynamic organization of complex neuronal systems. How much less informative, then, are the distant reflections of neural events which can be recorded from electrical spaces on the human scalp? The apparent crudity of these data is, however, misleading. In Dr. Vaughan's view, human brain potentials can, with proper analytic treatment, yield information concerning the spatial and temporal pattern of brain activity during behavior which can be obtained in no other way.

In man alone can one explore the complexity of language perception and of short term cognitive processes and retrieval from memory in relation to their underlying physiological mechanisms. The questions which may be asked of these electrical data concern where and when brain actions occur in relation to specific psychological processes. These data bring under empirical examination Von Monakov's concept of chronological localization of function within the brain.

Virtually all current information of functional specialization of brain regions is derived from observations of the effects of cerebral lesions or electrical stimulation supplemented by as yet incomplete anatomical knowledge of regional neural interconnections. These data are very important but provide no information concerning the extent of the neural systems involved in a specific behavioral pattern or of the temporal sequence of activity in relevant structures. This information is critical to the formulation of dynamic system models of brain function.

During the past decade, Dr. Vaughan's laboratory has worked to devise approaches to the analysis of human brain physiology which can provide reliable data about chronological functional localization. The averaging method for extracting time-locked signals from the EEG permits the detection of what Dr. Vaughan has designated as "event-related potentials," synchronized by external stimuli or by other identifiable events.

Workers in this laboratory have been successful in showing that all of these waveforms, which are transients, last about a quarter of a second in total duration from the first indication of response of the cortex to the evident termination of these processes. They have been able to show that these elementary sensory evoked responses are generated in and near the primary projection areas of the human cortex known primarily from anatomical data.

In addition to the sensory evoked responses which are extracted from the EEG by averaging with respect to the presentation of the number of identical stimuli, one can also extract from the EEG activity related to voluntary movement. In 1963, Drs. Gilden and Vaughan were successful, by averaging with respect to a repeated voluntary motor contraction, in recording from the precentral region potentials which anteceded the muscle contraction and were concomitant with the burst of muscle activity. They have shown in monkeys that similar potentials can be recorded from the surface of the cortex; the waveform of the gross surface motor potential in monkeys correlates very closely with the histogram of parameter unit activity which occurs in association with a trained hand movement. There is thus a good relationship, in this particular instance, between the firing pattern of the pyramidal tract neuron in the underlying cortex and the surface potential recorded from the cortical surface.

The recording of these stimulus-and-response-related potentials makes it possible to analyze a number of sensorimotor processes which can be very simple or extraordinarily complex — involving cognitive processes, memory retrieval, and language. Using these tools, events are being studied that occur in different parts of the brain during increasingly complex psychological processes.

Drs. Ritter and Vaughan, in studying habituation of evoked responses in human subjects, found that when a stimulus was presented unexpectedly a large wave of considerably longer latency than the ordinary sensory response appeared. Subsequently, they have shown that this activity is present whenever a stimulus is used as sensory information. The source of this late wave has been found to be distinct from that of the sensory evoked potentials; it arises in the parietal-temporal cortex. Dr. Vaughan and his co-workers call these waveforms "association cortex potentials."

These investigators have also worked extensively on the problem of identifying intracranial sources of scalp potentials and have attempted to estimate the strength of the equivalent intracranial generators. They have succeeded in developing what they believe to be a reasonable volume conductor model of the brain and its covering. With this model, empirically derived amplitude distributions of potentials recorded under specified behavioral conditions can be compared with theoretical distributions conforming to hypothetical intracranial sources of specified size, location, and configuration.

The hypothesis concerning the intracranial source geometry to date is based largely on anatomical knowledge of cortical projections. Dr. Vaughan and his co-workers have found a good fit between the empirical data and the reasonable hypotheses one might make about the source of potentials, including the relationship between the measured amplitude of the evoked potentials recorded intracranially and the amplitude recorded from the scalp surface. These workers therefore feel that this model can be used as a means to define further the sources of potentials associated with more complex behaviors.

Dr. Vaughan and his co-workers are currently constructing a physiological map of cortical organization of sensorimotor sequences. They have already done this for the visual-, activity-, and somatosensory-evoked potentials; for the motor potentials; and for the long latency association cortex potentials.

Experiments now in progress are analyzing the cerebral potentials related to the most complex system yet studied: the control of eye movements. In this investigation, subjects are required to execute carefully controlled voluntary saccadic eye movements. The potentials associated with these movements are time-locked to the onset of each eye movement. They consist of two distinct sets of potentials: one which begins before and another which follows the eye movement. These potentials can be distinguished from one another both temporally and spatially.

The potentials which follow the eye movement (called "lambda waves") have been shown to be essentially responses evoked by movement of a patterned visual field across the retina. These are generated in the occipital visual cortex. The antecedent potentials show two loci of potential: one over the precentral region and the other over the parieto-occipital cortex.

What are the implications of these methods for study of the developing human brain? By means of these mapping techniques it is now possible to obtain functional maturational maps of the cortical areas which Dr. Vaughan and his co-workers have identified physiologically in the adult and are exploring in more detail in the subhuman primate. Of particular interest will be the development of the parieto-temporal association area, in view of the likely implication of these areas in the development of intermodal interactions, language, and other aspects of cognitive functioning. It is likely that crude, but reliable indices of some cortical processes related to the more complex psychological processes may be reached in the foreseeable future.

Dr. Vaughan raised some of the problems which confront this work. First, the relationship is unknown between these gross potentials (whether recorded from the scalp, from the cortical surface, or from gross electrodes within the cerebral tissue itself) and the underlying cellular patterns of activity. The relationship between EEG activity and cellular firing patterns has not been resolved, in part because it has not been a very interesting problem for neurophysiologists. It is, however, an important problem for behavioral physiology, since there are serious limitations to studies using chronic microelectrode recording in the behaving animal. Among these limitations must be mentioned the inherent sampling bias involved in the microelectrode method, as well as the great difficulty of obtaining simultaneous single-unit data from several structures within a functional system. The latter requirement must be met in order to define a temporal pattern of neural activity related to a given behavioral sequence.

According to Dr. Vaughan, the gross potential technique has the advantage of being a rather sensitive method for determining the timing and presence of over-all neural activity in a particular structure (although unrevealing as to the precise cellular pattern of firing). It requires, however, that one have a clear picture of the field of the particular potential under consideration. This factor has not received sufficient attention in human brain potential studies.

There is a pressing need to consider further the relationship between gross potentials and unit activity in behaving animals. A number of studies deal principally with spontaneous EEG rhythm and responses to electrical stimulation (recruiting responses, augmenting responses). The pattern of neural activity during behavior may be quite different from that generated by electrical stimulation of the thalamus or in anesthetized animals. While this may be a rather obvious point, it is one which Dr. Vaughan believes now urgently needs empirical resolution.

The EEG has not been discussed mainly because the problems of relating spontaneous cerebral activity to behavior are fairly well known. There has been a good deal of effort expended on the problems of the statistical analysis of the EEG using computational methods, and it is well known that the EEG power spectra change during alterations in arousal level. However, in Dr. Vaughan's view, while analysis of the spontaneous electrical activity of the brain cannot be forgotten in any study which extracts signals from it, it seems to be a blunter tool than the study of event-related potentials. It is still unfeasible to extract from the ongoing pattern of electrical activity correlations between complex behavior and electrical patterns. An artificial temporal patterning must be imposed upon brain processes to relate a physiological activity to the experiential and behavioral variables.

Behavioral validation of these measures is also needed in gross evoked potential studies. To Dr. Vaughan, it is not desirable to wait until physiologists eventually demonstrate how different classes of neurons in striate cortex are related to the various components of visual evoked responses. Understanding of the physiological mechanisms underlying experience and behavior may be more readily advanced by establishing quantitative relationships between psychological variables and gross measures of brain activity along the lines suggested by Dr. Vaughan.

Dr. Vaughan and his co-workers have been successful, in a number of experiments, in showing a quantitative correlation between psychophysical measures such as brightness or spectral sensitivity and changes in visual evoked response. With still further correlations, it should be possible to suggest the direction for more detailed analysis in experimental animals.

# SESSION IV.
# DEVELOPMENT OF COGNITIVE FUNCTIONS

# Introduction

H. Birch

Before dealing substantively with the problem of cognitive function, Dr. Birch related his own approach to some of the problems presented in the previous sessions. He noted that in Session III, several interesting and important findings were presented with respect to the development of the nervous system at the molecular level of organization. Included were descriptions of particular model systems relating to the growth of explants of the nervous system, discussions of the use of certain types of tumor models and cell systems for viewing aspects of CNS growth, and presentations concerning aspects of central nervous system biochemistry. All of this work, according to Dr. Birch, is of fundamental importance and in the long run cannot but contribute significantly to greater understanding of the central nervous system, its laws of growth, and its mechanisms of operation. Dr. Birch observed, however, that at the present stage of knowledge, the problems with which these investigators have been concerned and the issues they have explored are unintegrated with the issues of the central nervous system as a functional system mediating the individual organism's behavioral transactions with its environment.

It is at present extremely difficult to identify which of these investigations and sets of findings provide one with a clearer understanding of the manner in which the nervous system works to mediate behavior. Dr. Birch noted that at the current level of technological development it is unfair to ask that these same investigators provide an explanation of the mechanisms of behavior. Hopefully at some later point in time, findings at the molecular level may be integrated with more directed findings and investigations concerning the functions of the nervous system underlying and mediating behavioral organization. A fuller picture of the way in which the system works at a variety of organizational levels will then become available.

Scientists concerned with behavior deal with events at the supramolar level of central nervous system organization. Those concerned with cellular, subcellular, and molecular features of growth deal primarily with the lowest levels of organization of the system: at the level of biophysics or biochemistry. In Dr. Birch's view, the present stage of work, with some investigators studying behavior and others analyzing molecular organization of the central nervous system, may be characterized as what in child psychology is called "parallel play." That is to say, while research activity is based upon a common geography of concern, molecular and behavioral researchers are behaving quite independently of one another, each following laws of his own and relating to the other without mutual identification of shared scientific problems or issués. Such parallel relationships can at times be intriguing and may even at certain points raise a number of questions of possible immediacy of interrelationships. Dr. Birch believes that in the long run, however, the research endeavor should progress from parallel to integrated approaches. An understanding of the nervous system's functions and the laws of its functioning can occur only by stating problems which can be investigated in common.

In introducing the subsequent substantive materials of Session IV, Dr. Birch formulated certain kinds of questions in the development of behavior which he hopes may facilitate movement from the stage of disciplinary parallelism into one of interaction. He noted that it may be grossly unfair for a behavioral scientist to make demands upon molecular biologists and neurophysiologists. Yet such demands are based on the belief that the origins of neurophysiology in the work of Sherrington, for example, derive precisely from efforts to define behaviors which can be accounted for by features of organization and integration in the nervous system.

The models used and the questions asked by behavioral scientists vary widely. Thus, one of the ways in which people have tended to view the origins of behavioral development and the nature of initial behavioral organization is by considering behaviors to be divisible and organized into discrete stimulus-response relationships in which the application of a particular stimulus produces a particular action upon the part of the organism. In other words, one view of the primary behavioral process is reflexive. The nervous system is believed to be so organized that an energy input through a receptor results in a particular and defined output through some effector organization. For people who hold strongly to this reflexive view, the development of behavior represents the accumulation of such reflexes, the development of chains of association among individual reflex elements, and, as a result of these additive processes, the creation of new complexity in organization. They view a complex act such as locomotion as the extension of a series of part reflexes related to reflexes of limbs, to the orientation of the head in response to visual stimulation, and to certain postural adjustments in relation to gravity. The development of the act of walking is seen as the addition of these reflexes to one another in a particular sequence and order.

In Dr. Birch's opinion, if one views behavioral development in this way, one can demand of neurophysiologists answers to the following questions: 1) Is there a mechanism for such independent reflex organization? 2) By what mechanism do individual reflexes become able to combine with one another to create sequences and patterns? What kind of behavioral development and organization needs to be mediated?

This particular model of behavioral organization is less attractive to Dr. Birch than an alternative which he subsequently discussed. He observed that in examining very young organisms (a fetus or a newborn), one finds isolated single responses under particular experimental circumstances. Yet under other conditions, one sees diffuseness in the expression of activity by any organism. As the organism grows older and its structure and functions alter over time, responsiveness gradually becomes more explicit. In other words, the organism may be viewed as being initially both highly differentiated and relatively undifferentiated with respect to its processing of information inputs. Information processing subsequently becomes increasingly explicit, and differentiation of action occurs in association with the development of particular organizations of behavior.

To Dr. Birch, such a view makes it possible to place a different demand upon the neurophysiologist. Instead of asking him which mechanism can, in fact, account for association between independent reflexes, one may now ask him why at one age and state a stimulus results in widespread and diffuse manifestations of behavior and at others in explicit responding. What are the changes at the physiological, the biochemical, or anatomical levels that result in the constriction of response? To ask this question focuses attention upon a newly developing and highly active and growing area of research in electrophysiology—namely, the organization of inhibition rather than of excitation, and the development of mechanisms through which selective organization of inhibition may, in fact, take place.

Thus, by looking at early behavior and its development in different ways, a behavioral scientist might make different demands upon his colleagues in the more molecular areas of investigation and might pose different questions to them. He might then ask: What is known with respect to the organization and growth of the nervous system at the molecular level which can account for explicitness in expression of organization, in the phenomena of differentiation, or in the developing phenomena of inhibition and selective inhibition?

Dr. Birch believes that by beginning to pose such questions, it will be possible to move from areas in which parallelism is being exhibited into areas in which discussions are about common concerns and problems. One can thus define common issues for investigation and work.

The process and the problem become even more complex if one looks at behavior and its development and organization in a slightly broader way, according to Dr. Birch. Within the behavioral sciences over the past 20 to 25 years, there has been an enormous growth of interest in an approach to analyzing behavior which has been characterized as "ethology."

Years ago, work in this area was called "animal behavior." Dr. Birch reports that the term "ethology" replaced "animal behavior" or "the behavior of organisms" because biologists preferred its Greek sound. However, as he noted, ethology is not merely the study of the behavior of organisms; it is a point of view. It is a conceptualization of behavior which argues that at every species level, built into the structure of the nervous system, there are specific, geographically localized, organized patterns of neuronal integration. Further, it argues that the basic behaviors of a species are not the result of responses to stimuli. Rather, they represent the projection out upon the world of intrinsically organized activities of the central nervous system arising from some kind of internal energy accumulation. In other words, behavior is believed to be spontaneously expressed independently of explicit stimulation, in accordance with the condensed energy that has somehow or other accumulated within the nervous system itself.

Dr. Birch questioned whether biologists who have become very accepting of ethological notions have explored the implications of this concept for neurophysiology. What does it demand of the neurophysiologists? Clearly, at the level of the anatomical organization, much more information is needed about the explicit anatomical organization of act sequences and patterns. At another level, it demands of the neurophysiologist and the neurochemist some mechanism for explicit localized energy accumulation, i.e., specific act energy accumulations, within the central nervous system.

What are the mechanisms, if any, of condensation and storage of energy within regions of the central nervous system? Is the entire concept of behavioral organization a myth which has no basis in neurophysiological organization and poses no explorable problem at the level of molecular investigation of the nervous system? These are very serious questions in general biology that Dr. Birch, as a behavioral scientist, poses to the students of the molecular organization of the central nervous system.

There are still other problems in behavior. For example, in the study of children and their development, individual differences in behavioral development are frequently noted. Such differences are most dramatically manifested between mentally retarded and normally developing children. One of the ways of identifying processes of behavioral organization is the comparative analysis of handicapped and normally developing children. In the latter, with increasing age there is a growing capacity of the organism to process simultaneously multisensory information from the environment. The individual is able to integrate information across sensory systems and to treat information from one sense system as equivalent to information from another. For example, by 6 or 7 years of age, a child is able to identify whether or not an auditory temporal sequence is the same as or different from a like temporal sequence presented visually.

Normal children exhibit a beautifully developing course of intersensory equivalents and of intersensory competence. However, children whose brains are damaged, or children who are developing defectively, or who have been insulted, for example, by extensive degrees of malnutrition in the course of their development, exhibit significant deficiencies in their ability to process such information across sensory systems. Obviously, the ability to engage in such processing is critical for one's ability to learn to read, to write, and to engage in a whole series of complex behaviors and skills.

Behavioral scientists need to learn from molecular biologists which changes underlie these shifts. What type of nervous system organization results in a relative independence of sense systems in information processing early in the development of the organism? What are the processes of change (anatomical, physiological, and biochemical) which permit the development of information processing between sensory systems?

A beginning can be made, in Dr. Birch's opinion, by looking at both the initial organization of behavior and the course of change in behavioral organizations with growth. One can then identify those behavioral problems of change and of organization whose solution requires fuller physiological and anatomical understanding. Analyses such as these hopefully can create a basis for developing useful cross-communication between the student of behavior and the student of the molecular organization of the nervous system.

Dr. Birch observed that in the final analysis all molecular understanding of nervous system organization will have as its ultimate test the degree to which it permits one to explain how the system performs its functional role—namely, the mediation of behavioral organizations.

# Development of Infant Behavior

**L. Lipsitt**

Dr. Lipsitt began his presentation by observing that inviting him to speak on the development of cognitive structures in infants is somewhat like inviting an agnostic to preach a sermon in church on Sunday. He does not really believe in cognitive structure; to him the expression "cognitive structure" is metaphorical. As in a number of other instances in which terms have been appropriated gratuitously from the field of biology to account for behavior, there is a great possibility that the theoretical use of a "cognitive-structural" concept will distort the behavioral observations from which the "structural" inferences are made. The postulation of "stages" to represent plateaus of behavior and to connote that at different ages different behavioral adjustments seem most appropriate may have some heuristic and abbreviatory value. However, as Dr. Lipsitt warned, some scientists tend to reify such hypothetical constructs, then act observationally, theoretically, and linguistically as if these stages were essentially immutable. The use of stage concepts, stage theories, and inferred "cognitive structures" may, in other words, help the observer to *organize* the observed behavior, but in Dr. Lipsitt's view, it should be understood that cognitive organization is more in the beholder than in the behaver.

Unfortunately, stage-restriction theories tend to forestall certain types of empirical investigation. If one believes, for example, that the 3-year-old child is not ready to read, then one will not investigate the processes and limits of reading age. One will thus not explore techniques for learning to read, and the reading readiness concept will have been gratuitously supported. The appropriation of the reading readiness concept by educationists from the field of child development has, in Dr. Lipsitt's opinion, had a stultifying effect upon research into the processes and mechanisms by which reading behavior comes about.

Dr. Lipsitt noted that his remarks are not to be taken as a denial of reductionism. In his view, all behavior is mediated through the organism's nervous system, and without question the nervous system consists of structures. Indeed, if one does not believe in the nervous system mediation of behavior, one must then believe in ghosts. The reductionistic stand does not, however, demand the postulation of cognitive structures. Indeed, in Dr. Lipsitt's opinion, cognitive structure does not have any known physical representation in the nervous system.

Dr. Lipsitt cited what he called "an excellent example of the manner in which the premature postulation of structural limitations may have an inhibiting effect upon behavioral research," using an example drawn from the history of research into conditioning processes of infants. For many years it has been known that myelination is absent or grossly under-developed in the very young primate. When some of the early conditioning studies in human infants failed to demonstrate learning, researchers often resorted to the explanation that underdevelopment of myelinization was responsible. Resorting to such a "structural" explanation helped to exonerate the research failure and made it seem futile to investigate further other behavioral events that might have been more conducive to elaborating a learning process. Naturally, there are congenital limitations to the conditionability of any organism, including the newborn human. However, as Dr. Lipsitt observed, it should not have been a foregone conclusion that any given conditioning failure was justifiably attributable to a structural limitation. The history of conditioning in the young infant has since yielded the insight that perseverance in behavioral methodology and technology can produce learning. All conditioning depends in fact upon congenital *permissions*, but one can only know the extent of those permissions when the appropriate experiential conditions have enabled them to operate. According to Dr. Lipsitt, it is thus inappropriate, for example, to assume that early education is not beneficial just because "Head Start" (whatever complicated antecedent condition that term represents) did not succeed in appreciably facilitating the education of some youngsters.

For the past 12 years or so, Dr. Lipsitt and his co-workers have been studying the behavioral processes of newborns and older infants using a wide variety of techniques designed to explore the plasticity of infant behavior. The studies, which have been conducted in their laboratories at the Providence Lying-In Hospital and at a local orphanage, have enabled them to draw a picture of the developing infant's behavior which suggests that the newborn child is remarkably more precocious than has traditionally been appreciated.

Dr. Lipsitt described the methods used to record sucking, respiration, heart rate, stabilimeter activity, and other response processes in the newborn. He and his associates have shown that the sucking behavior of the newborn is remarkably orderly, and that parameters derived from sucking behavior permit the close study of, for example, reinforcement-contrast phenomena. Newborns suck more to receive sucrose than to receive water, and when sucking for water during a period following sucrose-sucking activity, the water-sucking rate is depressed. After testing the newborns' sense of smell, these workers showed that habituation of response takes place, followed by recovery of response when an alternative olfactory stimulus is introduced. Dr. Lipsitt presented data showing that newborns can learn a head-turning discrimination within 30 minutes and can then be shown to engage in a discrimination reversal. Data were also presented which indicate that eyelid conditioning can readily occur in infants as young as 10 days of age, provided the appropriate interstimulus interval is used.

# The Detection of Brain Dysfunction in the Newborn Infant

**G. Turkewitz**

Many concerned with the development of normal and abnormal functioning are dissatisfied with the limited extent to which current techniques permit abnormal functioning to be identified very early in life. Although severely damaged newborns are easily recognized, lesser degrees of impairment frequently escape detection with standard methods of clinical assessment.

Almost a quarter of a century ago Monnier and Willie demonstrated that, with the exception of the visual following response, reflex organization is grossly normal, even in anencephalic infants. According to Dr. Turkewitz, it is, therefore, obvious that if sensitive techniques are to be developed for the early identification of handicap, one must go beyond standard examinations of reflex organization and direct attention to more complex neural behavior.

A number of alternative strategies have been used in an effort to increase diagnostic sensitivity. Workers such as Prechtl (1958) have sought to modify the pediatric neurological schedule to include factors such as tonus and lateral equality as well as more standard reflexes in their examination of infant status. Other workers have approached the problem by examining electrophysiological measures ranging from EEG, through sleep patterns, to evoked cortical responses. There has as yet been little attempt to identify atypical infants on the basis of their learning ability. However, Dr. Turkewitz believes that the recent development and application of elegant techniques such as Dr. Lipsitt's will undoubtedly encourage exploration of this approach in the near future. Each of these approaches has its own merit and should, therefore, be pressed.

There are certain limitations, however, attached to each of them. Since investigation of infant reflexes and muscle tonus normally includes little higher level function, such indicators are frequently quite insensitive to even marked neurological deficiencies. Although examining neuroelectrical activity is a promising method for identifying individuals with immature or defective neurointegrative organization, it is limited by imperfect understanding of the way such neurophysiological activity relates to behavior.

A relationship between maturation of EEG activity and learning capacity is suggested, if one considers together the finding that the EEG alpha rhythm of puppies does not appear until they are 3 weeks old, as well as the discovery by Fuller et al. (1950) that puppies could not be conditioned until they were 3 weeks of age. In more recent findings, however, it has been shown that under appropriate conditions, learning could be accomplished by puppies during the 1st week of life, that is, while the EEG pattern is still quite immature. In Dr. Turkewitz' view, this raises serious questions about the nature of the relationship between EEG findings and neurointegrative organization.

Similarly, it has been shown that infant rats exhibiting precocial patterns of evoked potentials show a depression in certain types of learning at later ages. This indicates to Dr. Turkewitz that assessments of neurointegrative integrity based upon the appearance of electrocortical events are at the present time on shaky ground. When thyroxin was administered to infant rats, they showed mature patterns of evoked potentials. However, when the same animals were tested at older ages, they also showed certain deficits in learning.

Finally, although the study of learning during early infancy may well allow the detection of infants having problems during early life, the extensive time needed to investigate such learning may well make the technique prohibitive as a general indicator.

In view of these limitations, in Dr. Turkewitz' laboratory the strategy has been to attempt to identify behaviors that: 1) require a relatively high degree of integration; 2) can be exhibited by the infant without any special training; and 3) are potentially important for the future development of the infant.

Since many patterns of normal behavior, ranging from speech and reading to fine motor coordination, seem to require stable patterns of lateral differentiation, it appeared likely to these workers that lateralization of functioning during the neonatal period might represent a sensitive indicator of neurobehavioral organization and might be of more than minor importance for the subsequent organization of behavior. They therefore focused attention on identifying lateralized aspects of behavioral organization in the human newborn.

In selecting a particular aspect of lateral differentiation for study, certain principles of development were used as guides. It has long been recognized that a gradient of development occurs along the cephalocaudal axis such that development at the head end is more advanced than that of the trunk or extremities. It therefore seemed likely that those responses which occurred at or near the infant's head end would be more advanced than other responses, and that head-end responses, being of a higher level of organization, would represent maximally sensitive indicators of neurointegrative organization.

Attention was therefore concentrated on head-end responses of the infant: head-turning and eye-movement responses. Furthermore, very early in the search for organized behaviors in newborns, it became evident that directional responses to spatially distributed stimuli are among the earliest organized patterns of behavior to emerge in ontogeny.

The early emergence of such patterns is evidenced by their appearance in the embryo, fetus, and neonate of such diverse vertebrate forms as salamanders, rats, cats, and guinea pigs. In view of their prevalence and early appearance, directionalized behaviors appear to Dr. Turkewitz to represent a potential source of sensitive indicators of neurointegrative organization.

The principal strategy of Dr. Turkewitz and his co-workers has, therefore, been to look for such indicators among the laterally differentiated directional responses of the infant's head end, specifically lateral differences in the infant's head-turning response to laterally applied somesthetic stimulation of the perioral region. Using this indicator, infants whose developmental history has been unexceptional are compared with infants whose histories suggest that they are at an elevated risk of neurointegrative disturbances.

Dr. Lipsitt pointed out that when newborns are touched at the corner of the mouth, they tend to turn in the direction of such stimulation. Dr. Turkewitz' laboratory has found, however, that although the prevalent response to tactile stimulation is a turn in the direction of the stimulus, the response is more readily elicited when the infant is stimulated on the right side of the face than on the left. Similarly, although contralateral responses are infrequent, they occur more frequently when the stimulus is applied to the left side than to the right. Thus, there appears to be a typical pattern of lateral differentiation: the infant is more responsive to tactile stimulation to the right than to the left.

Having identified an early-appearing pattern of lateral differentiation in normal infants, Dr. Turkewitz compared the patterns of lateral differentiation among infants who had different degrees of exposure to conditions associated with later manifestations of central nervous system damage.

Although infants in suboptimal condition at birth frequently appeared to recover by the end of 2 days, they exhibited a relatively high frequency of abnormalities in motor, language, and intellectual functioning during later infancy and childhood. It therefore appeared possible to Dr. Turkewitz and his associates that the effects of poor conditions at birth would not be evanescent, and that there would be a continuing disorganization which was merely masked by the insensitivity of routine clinical investigation.

To explore this possibility, the research team compared 2-day-old infants who had been in poor condition at birth (but who according to routine clinical investigation had completely recovered by the time they were seen), and control infants whose condition at birth and thereafter was good. Those infants who were in poor condition at birth were found to make head turns as frequently as normal controls. However, there were marked differences in the lateral differentiation of these responses. As a group, those infants who had been in poor condition at birth did not turn toward the right more frequently than toward the left. As is always the case, not all of these infants exhibited an atypical pattern of lateral differentiation. However, even those infants who were more responsive to stimulation of the right than left exhibited such differentiation to a lesser extent than normal controls.

These findings suggest either that the recovery of the initially suboptimal infants was more apparent than real, or that the early malfunctioning had contributed during the perinatal period to a sequence of development which led to establishment of atypical patterns of lateral differences.

To Dr. Turkewitz and his co-workers, it is obvious that examining early lateral differentiation represents a useful approach to identifying infants with exceptional neurointegrative organization. In their view it is likely that lateral differentiation or its absence during the early postnatal period affects subsequent development. However, the relationship between early lateral differentiation and subsequent functioning must be examined before one can assume that the disturbance of lateral differentiation observed in the young infant is related to the variety of functional disabilities and associated laterality disturbances found in older children and adults.

Members of Dr. Turkewitz' laboratory have conducted a series of investigations into some of the factors underlying the normal pattern of lateral differentiation. They hope that eventually specific mechanisms can be isolated which might be affected in those infants showing atypical patterns of lateral differentiation.

Dr. Turkewitz has found that newborns in nurseries typically lie with their heads turned to the right. In this position, they receive unequal stimulation at the two sides. Lateral differences in auditory stimulation are produced because the mattress occludes one ear, resulting in less stimulation at one side than at the other; lateral differences in tactile stimulation also result from the infant's contact with the mattress.

Dr. Turkewitz and his co-workers thought these differences in input might be crucial to early lateral differentiation. To test this, the baby was prevented from being exposed to lateral differences in input (by having its head held in the midline position for 15 minutes) just prior to testing for lateral differentiation in either tactile or auditory responsiveness.

When this was done, the left-right differences in responsiveness to both auditory and tactile stimulation were effectively eliminated. Since the association between prior head position and subsequent lateral differences in responsiveness might have derived from differences either in sensory input or in muscle tonus associated with the asymmetrical head position, the following investigation which included four groups of infants was conducted.

One group of infants had their heads held in the midline with no additional stimulation (the absence of lateral differentiation both in tonus or input). Two groups had their heads in the midline, but had somesthetic input applied in one case to the right side and in the other to the left side. Infants in the fourth group had a lateral difference in tonus induced by holding their heads to the right. In this latter group, lateral differences in somesthetic input were prevented by not allowing contact between the infants' heads and the substrate.

Under these conditions, the results were as expected: the control group (the group with its head held in the midline with no stimulation) exhibited no left-right difference in responsiveness. The tonus group (the group with the head held to the right) exhibited the usual right-left difference: more responsiveness to stimulation at the right than the left. The group held in the midline, but given somesthetic prestimulation at the right side was also more responsive to stimulation at the right than left.

The major unexpected finding was that infants prestimulated at the left were not more responsive to stimulation at the left than at the right—in fact, they were slightly more responsive to stimulation at the right, suggesting that whatever had been done at the right and left sides was not equivalent. There is therefore another factor to be considered. Either as a result of the baby's preceding history of lying on one side or as a result of whatever produced the initial propensity to lie on one side, there is an inequality in the effect which stimulation at the two sides will exert on subsequent lateral differentiation.

# Toward a Strategy of Analysis of Behavioral Development

**G. Meier**

According to Dr. Meier, overt, measurable behavior is the interaction of an organism and its environment by which both the organism and the environment are progressively changed. The character of these interactions, that is, the qualitative and quantitative aspects of a given organism's behavioral repertoire, are intrinsically related to its species and other taxonomic considerations, its age, its sex, and the peculiar past and present social-physical aspects of its environment. The ontogeny of behavior (the pattern of development of that behavior which is clearly related to each of these dimensions of analysis) is that particular aspect of development whereby the interaction becomes more complex and diverse and the repertoire of behavior progressively expands and becomes more elaborate. In this communication process, both the media and the messages become increasingly enriched — while the possibilities for alteration progressively contract in the face of no fundamental change in the variety and number of environmental opportunities available. In short, in the careful description of the growth of the behavioral repertoire of a single individual, one sees the selfsame processes imputed to the evolution of the species: progressive use of opportunities offered by the environment (i.e., "ecological niches"), increasing specialization of the evolutionary line, and increasingly fine adaptation to the environmental contingencies, with concurrent loss of flexibility should those opportunities be suddenly and dramatically altered.

Dr. Meier underscored the "truism" that the organism does not exist in a vacuum naturally and should not be compelled to do so scientifically in the name of "analysis and control." The behavior of the individual organism is one facet of its being in which this organism-environment dyad is seen immediately, if not most clearly. Moreover, if an interaction truly exists (and Dr. Meier believes most would concur that it does), then new approaches must be sought in which one can look at that particular relationship where cause and effect become intertwined (and therefore confused) and where the application of nice dichotomies like *independent variable* and *dependent variable* became heuristically and systematically meaningless. One must turn to a methodology of investigation whereby ontogeny can be viewed as a process and not as a series of discrete points, stages, or periods, critical or otherwise.

In Dr. Meier's view, each investigator designs his own test tube; each devises his own model of the reality of life and the means whereby he can study the particular life phenomena to which his interest is most acutely drawn and his talents best suited. Dr. Meier has elected to look at infant-caretaker relations in primates from a period shortly after birth to some time thereafter, even to the eventual establishment of the next generation. Some advantages of such a model system are immediately obvious: a time-base relatively consistent with our own, with ample occasion to observe the detail of behavioral growth; behavioral characteristics sufficiently similar to our own behavioral concerns; characteristics of social organization, from the usual single births to the usual matriarchal family organization with a heavy overlay of super-familial social hierarchy suggestive of our basic societies; the opportunity for uninterrupted continuity of observation over extended periods, even over full generations. Obviously this orientation also presents serious disadvantages: the advanced (i.e., neonatal) developmental age at outset; the tediousness and laboriousness of data collection over such extended periods that descriptions of interactions are slow in evolving; the deluge of data which seemingly defy reduction; the propensity to anthropomorphize to other primates and vice versa; and the complex interactions between individual target infants, caretakers, and other individuals in such a manner that all are grossly or subtly confounded.

These are concerns and approaches at the conceptual-methodological level. At the technical level, Dr. Meier advocates the application of those constant or chronic monitoring procedures long successful in the single subject technology of the experimental analysis of behavior. He acknowledged at present that the application of this level of involvement in the developmental process has not been achieved — and the hope of even limited success in the very near future is dim, indeed. Nevertheless, progress in allied fields such as experimental surgery, computer technology, telemetry, biomedical instrumentation, and primate care and management, for example, encourages him to believe that that hope can be fulfilled in a reasonable period, providing the effort is given continued support and enlightened understanding.

Two research problems were cited by Dr. Meier which illustrate the application of the approach he has advocated. The first deals with the sequelae of neonatal brain damage as inflicted by a bout of asphyxiation or by experimental manipulation in the form of electrolytic or surgical lesions. Animals so prepared present serious problems of detection; few aftereffects resemble those anticipated on the basis of a model of generalized developmental or mental retardation.

The second deals with the long range effects of essential isolation during infancy. Although all agree that such animals, especially monkeys, are bizarre in their behavior (usually prone to stereotypes and other autisms), consensus has not been reached as to the effect on novelty-seeking and reproductive behaviors or on complex learning performances. Contrary to the postasphyxial sequelae, the behaviors of these animals are markedly different from mother- and peer-raised infants and suggest a very complex relation between developmental history and the conditions of behavioral assay.

Clarity can be achieved in both of these problem areas, according to Dr. Meier, if one analyzes the day-to-day, situation-to-situation interactions of the target infants and relates functionally the infants' characteristics with those of their environment. Such an analysis should reveal that certain behaviors will appear, will be followed (or not followed) by predictable environmental contingencies, and will increase (or decrease) accordingly. Changes in quantitative aspects of the developing organisms' behavioral repertoire will provide a basis for estimating the presence or absence of behavioral sequelae of neonatal brain damage. It should also be possible to predict the environmental circumstances which evoke the approach and withdrawal behaviors of the isolate-reared animal. Thus, a functional or contingent analysis must replace the cause-and-effect methodology so typical of comparative research on mental retardation.

If the infant is the sole concern (rather than the fetus), then more attention should be given to the manner and means whereby he maintains contact with his environment than to theoretical formulations of a presumed cognitive structure. As Dr. Meier observed, for survival, the mammalian infant *will* maintain contact; the environment *will* maintain contact with him. In this arena, behavioral development proceeds to adequate adult adaptation.

In summary, Dr. Meier noted that mental retardation does not exist in an aberrant cell, a confused intercellular configuration, or a unique biochemical, be it endocrinal or metabolic. It does, instead, result from a prolonged series of interactions between an organism which is more-or-less responsive and an environment which is more-or-less stimulating. Heretofore, only the result has been studied, and causal relations have been assumed from correlations. It is time to look at the process, recognize the evolutionary character of mental retardation, and, eventually, realize the hope of modifying the course of events for the individual child of high risk.

# The Present State of Knowledge and Available Techniques in the Area of Cognition

S. Escalona

As Dr. Escalona observed in her final commentary on the symposium, the primary concern of the participants has been the study of human development in a neurobiological frame of reference. She noted that there have been implications that overt behavior, in this case cognitive behavior, rests upon neurophysiological structures and functions. All participants share scientific curiosity about developmental processes on all levels and are eager to discover the pathways and the mechanisms through which neurobiological events determine cognitive development. Dr. Escalona commented that most of the papers provided elegant examples of developmental studies within a narrow area, from the single neuron, through neonatal response patterns, to conditioning techniques. In addition, according to Dr. Escalona, Dr. Birch posed a series of fascinating questions concerned with possible links between biochemical or neural processes, on the one hand, and cognitive behavioral developments, on the other. In discussing the present state of knowledge and of available techniques in the area of cognition, Dr. Escalona observed that an adequate description, measurement, or comprehension of cognitive development is still far from realized. She sees many obstacles to the pursuit of the type of research inquiry outlined by Dr. Birch — at least for some time to come.

In her view, had this symposium been held 12 years ago, the word "intelligence" would have been used instead of "cognition." The change in terminology arose from dissatisfaction with the notion that a group of diverse and constantly changing functions can profitably be regarded as an entity or trait which individuals possess to a particular degree. The referent term "cognitive organization" implies that attention is given to more than the ability to perform successfully a finite number of particular tasks, as tested by standard intelligence tests. Instead, cognition is viewed as one variety of adaptive behavior, guided in part by central regulatory mechanisms that manifest themselves in a variety of ways, depending upon both the context and the contents of the adaptive challenge to which cognitive operations are applied. Certain developmental psychologists, Dr. Escalona included, think of cognitive development in terms of the emergence, partial dissolution, and reformation of increasingly complex structures. The question before those concerned with cognitive research is whether current research strategy and practice conform to the more inclusive view of intellectual functioning denoted by the term "cognitive organization."

The prototypical investigation is one in which a set of biological (or for that matter socioenvironmental) variables are to be examined for their effects upon cognitive development. The "hypothesis" is that malnutrition, an enzyme deficiency, prematurity, or social class will show a correlation with the level or degree of cognitive ability. According to Dr. Escalona, such an expectation is not usually anchored to more particular hypotheses about the pathways or mechanisms that lead to the correlation. That is, one does not predict *which* aspects of cognitive development will be affected by *what* components of the physiological or environmental syndrome, nor the age at which the relationship is expected to emerge. Therefore, such studies really constitute two separate research enterprises converging upon the same subject population. Important empirical discoveries have been made in this manner. For instance, it is now known that paranatal complications, social class, and malnutrition are associated with lower levels of those types of intellectual performance especially important to academic achievement in Western schools (the varieties tapped by intelligence tests). However, these studies have not brought nearer an understanding of *how* malnutrition or any of the variables interact with cognitive behaviors.

Dr. Escalona noted that if one regards correlational studies of this sort as fishing expeditions, as cross-disciplinary rather than interdisciplinary studies, it is not to deprecate their merits but to define them as suited to fact finding and to the formulation of hypotheses—in contrast to validating types of research. Yet she believes that on occasion such research is planned, and research results reported as if available criterion measures were adequate and the relevant dimensions of cognitive phenomena had already been delineated.

Intelligence tests or a battery of standard cognitive tests addressed to specific functions are the most common techniques of assessing cognitive development. They are, in her opinion, the best tools currently available (at least if a quantitative measure is required) and may be well used provided that the limitations of these instruments are kept in mind. In other words, standard tests are designed to measure certain capacities such as memory, abstraction, form discrimination, and the like; this they do, within the narrow limits of the testing situation. Dr. Escalona warned, however, that failure to demonstrate these abilities in relation to particular tasks does not mean the same abilities cannot be demonstrated in other situations. Cross-cultural studies, including recent investigations of the mental function of ghetto children, have proven otherwise. For instance, some children who cannot solve a simple form-board problem can demonstrate incredibly fine form discrimination when it comes to the shape of leaves, or of ripples on the surface of water—if they happen to have grown up in an African fishing village. Similarly, the same juvenile delinquents who on testing showed marked deficit with respect to the functions of anticipation, planning, and capacity for delay manifested a high level of precisely these capacities when it came to the planning and execution of complex antisocial projects.

This is but one example of many lines of evidence to show that cognitive behavior is indivisible from motivation and from past life experience. One of the few things known about cognitive development is that learning takes place through the exercise of emerging functions, applied in the service of curiosity, of pleasure in mastery, of the need to escape distress, and of sheer survival. In consequence, even when the research design carefully controls not only the independent variable but also a series of others such as social class, ordinal position, or whatever, a large portion of the variance in cognitive function-ing remains unexplained. Conventionally, this is handled by assuming that these so-called "error factors" are randomly distributed and will therefore "cancel out," so that group re-sults remain unaffected. Unfortunately, motivation and the life experiences that create it are not random in their distribution. For instance, a child whose early years of life were marked by frequent illness or by the aftermath of paranatal complications is—in addition to these direct impediments—subject to other problems such as emotional distress arising from a lack of bodily vigor and an unfavorable perception of the self. The same is true of malnourished children, who usually are also poor. In all likelihood, such children lack not only bodily and intellectual nourishment, but also the social and person-al supports that motivate them to take advantage of whatever learning opportunities do exist. Among psychologists such a premium is placed on reporting results that can be shown to be statistically significant that—since the techniques for establishing significance require random distribution—ran-domness is at times assumed when in fact there is evidence to the contrary.

Dr. Escalona believes that it is partly for this reason that reported differences in cognitive level are often so trivial. In the literature, I.Q. (or achievement score) differences of from 6 to 15 points are considered to be sizable. Yet except perhaps for extreme positions on the continuum, the practical con-sequences of functioning at an I.Q. level of 93 or 103 are negligible—not to speak of the fact that at least half of this difference is within the error range of the instrument. Accord-ing to Dr. Escalona, *statistical* significance at the 0.01 level simply has no bearing on the significance of the finding in social or in psychobiological terms.

Some major difficulties that beset research in cognitive development (especially when relationships to neurobiological development are sought for) were mentioned by Dr. Escalona.

The more ambitious cognitive studies are often longitu-dinal and obtain repeated measures of cognitive development over time. These tend to be reported in smoothed curves, reflecting the central tendency for each group. Yet as Dr. Escalona noted, anyone familiar with individual raw data

curves of intellectual development (such as those published by
MacFarlane and Bayley) knows that development tends to
proceed in irregular spurts, plateaus, and, not infrequently,
small dips. This is most prominent during the first 4 years, but
massive fluctuations can occur well into adolescence. Thus, for
any given measure at a given age, one never knows from the
group results what proportion of the subjects happened to be
caught at one of their peaks or one of their valleys.

A related issue is that once one gains access to the raw
data it can frequently turn out that within-group variations are
as large or larger than the difference between groups. Again
the conventions of research methodology and reporting can
mislead the unwary to believe that cognitive development and
its relationship to certain antecedents is more orderly than has
so far been actually demonstrated.

To Dr. Escalona, these and other sources of unreliability
and at times questionable validity of cognitive measures are
largely unavoidable: they reflect the state of the art. Yet, until
sharper tools have been developed, research results could be
used more productively if these shortcomings were more fully
recognized in the interpretation and reporting of results. For
instance, in the case of longitudinal studies, smoothed curves
reflecting central tendencies for groups could be supplemented by illustrative, uncorrected longitudinal data for individuals. It would be valuable to see all group differences
reported in such a way as to reflect the degree of overlap
between the groups (the standard deviation of the mean does
not necessarily reflect this). In fact, it would be helpful if the
practice of reporting the range and distribution separately for
each group became universal (it is now relatively rare), so that
the reader might compare within-group differences to
between-group differences.

One last issue raised by Dr. Escalona concerns instances
when a correlation between neurobiological and cognitive development has been established. One then knows the point in
time at which significant divergence from normal expectation
has occurred in cognitive development, as well as the timing
and the nature of the biological deficit or deviation. Even
under these happy circumstances, a causal link is difficult to
establish. It is true of cognition, as of other functions subject to
development, that the underlying process is continuous but

the overt manifestations (that is, cognitive behavior) are discontinuous. For instance, a new set of mental functions emerges when language is acquired. Nothing like verbal reasoning takes place before that time, yet Dr. Escalona's research and that of many others seeks to discover sensorimotor precursors of symbolic mental functioning. A similar qualitative break occurs later, somewhere during the 11th or 12th year, when entirely hypothetical reasoning (independent of information about and perception of reality) becomes possible. Therefore, a deficit in overt cognitive behavior may be related to concurrent bioneurological events or otherwise. It is just as logical to speculate that a decline observed at age 3 years is related to a deviance in neural integration that took place between 5 and 9 months of age, as to relate it to a concurrent biological event.

In conclusion, Dr. Escalona considers that multidisciplinary studies of nervous system development, insofar as they include cognitive development as one arm of the research, should be regarded as two or more parallel investigations. A detailed interlocking of neurobiological and cognitive phenomena in a developmental context seems to Dr. Escalona to be premature as yet.

She also believes that cognitive development needs to be studied in its own right and that such study will require experimental investigation of clusters of related functions over time. In other words, continued use of intelligence tests can have heuristic value but is not likely to contribute to greater understanding of cognition.

Each study related to cognitive development should be designed to stand on its own on psychological and behavioral grounds. Thus it can at the very least provide information about cognitive development. If the same sample is also studied in biological and other ways, so much the better; if suggestive correlations should emerge, new hypotheses may be formulated. Still, this is to be regarded as a bonus rather than a prime objective.

# Bibliography

Adinolfi, A. M., and Pappas, G. D. 1968. The fine structure of the caudate nucleus of the cat. J. Comp. Neurol. 133: 167.

Aghajanian, G. K., and Bloom, F. E. 1967. The formation of synaptic junctions in developing rat brain: A quantitative electron microscopic study. Brain Res. 6: 716.

Armstrong-James, M., and Johnson, R. 1970. Quantitative studies of postnatal changes in synapses in rat superficial motor cerebral cortex. An electron microscopical study. A. Zellforsch. Mikrosk. Anat. 110: 559.

Auerbach, A. A., and Bennett, M. V. L. 1969. Chemically mediated transmission at a giant fibre synapse in the central nervous system of a vertebrate. J. Gen. Physiol. 53: 183.

Bamburg, J. R., Reimer, K., and Wilson, L. 1971. Assay of microtubule protein in developing embryonic chick dorsal root ganglia. Fed. Proc. 30: 1194.

Barondes, S. H. 1967. Axoplasmic transport. A report of an NRP Work Session held April 2–4, 1967. Neurosci. Res. Prog. Bull. 5, 4: 307.

Barth, L. G., and Barth, L. J. 1969. The sodium dependence of embryonic induction. Develop. Biol. 20: 236.

Bennett, M. V. L., and Spira, M. E. 1971. Properties of junctions mediating electrical coupling between embryonic cells. Biol. Bull. 141: 378.

Bennett, M. V. L., and Trinkaus, J. P. 1970. Electric coupling between embryonic cells by way of extracellular space specialized junctions. J. Cell Biol. 44: 592.

Bennett, W. I., Gall, A. M., Southard, J. L., and Sidman, R. L. 1971. Abnormal spermiogenesis in quaking, a myelin-deficient mutant mouse. Biol. Reprod. 5: 30.

Bensch, K. G., and Malawista, S. E. 1968. Microtubule cyrstals: A new biophysical phenomenon induced by Vinca alkaloids. Nature (London) 218: 1176.

Bensch, K. G., and Malawista, S. E. 1969. Microtubular crystals in mammalian cells. J. Cell Biol. 40: 95.

Birks, R. I. 1971. Effects of stimulation on synaptic vesicles in sympathetic ganglia, as shown by fixation in the presence of Mg2+. J. Physiol. 216: 26[P.]

Borisy, G. G., and Taylor, E. W. 1967a. The mechanism of action of colchicine. Binding of colchicine-3H to cellular protein. J. Cell Biol. 34: 525.

Borisy, G. G., and Taylor, E. W. 1967b. The mechanism of action of colchicine. Colchicine binding to sea urchin eggs and mitotic apparatus. J. Cell Biol. 34: 535.

Bornstein, M. B. 1964. Morphological development of neonatal mouse cerebral cortex in tissue culture, p. 1. In P. Kellaway and I. Petersen (eds.), World Federation of Neurology. Neurological and electroencephalographic correlative studies in infancy. Grune and Stratton, New York.

Bornstein, M. B., and Crain, S. M. 1965. Functional studies of cultured brain tissues as related to demyelinative disorders. Science 148: 1242.

Bornstein, M. B., and Crain, S. M. 1971. Lack of correlation between changes in bioelectric functions and myelin in cultured CNS tissues chronically exposed to sera from animals with EAE. J. Neuropath. Exp. Neurol. 30: 129.

Bornstein, M. B., and Model, P. G. 1972. Development of synapses and myelin in cultures of dissociated embryonic mouse spinal cord, medulla and cerebrum. Brain Res. 37: 287.

Bornstein, M. B., and Murray, M. R. 1958. Serial observations on patterns of growth, myelin formation, maintenance and degeneration in cultures of new-born rat and kitten cerebellum. J. Biophys. Biochem. Cytol. 4, 5: 499.

Bornstein, M. B., and Raine, C. S. 1970. Experimental allergic encephalomyelitis. Antiserum inhibition of myelination in vitro. Lab. Invest. 23: 536.

Bornstein, M. B., and Raine, C. S. 1970. Experimental allergic encephalomyelitis. Inhibition of myelination and remyelination. Neurology 20: 389.

Bowen, D. M., and Radin, N. S. 1969. Cerebroside galactoside: A method for determination and a comparison with other lysosomal enzymes in developing rat brain. J. Neurochem. 16: 501.

Brown, R. E. 1966. Organ weight in malnutrition with special reference to brain weight. Develop. Med. Child. Neurol. 8: 512.

Bullock, T. H. 1967. Simple systems for the study of learning mechanisms. Neurosci. Res. Symp. Summ. 2: 203.

Bunge, M. B., Bunge, R. P., and Petersen, E. R. 1967. The onset of synapse formation in spinal cord cultures as studied by electron microscopy. Brain Res. 6: 728.

Burns, B. D. 1968. The uncertain nervous system. Edward Arnold, Ltd., London.

Carmichael, G. G. 1970. Application of the MTT-hydroquinone reaction in the study of hard tissue. J. Anat. 106: 194.

Carnegie, P. R. 1971. Properties, structure and possible neuroreceptor role of the encephalitogenic protein of human brain. Nature (London) 229: 25.

Changeux, J. P., Kasai, M., and Lee, C. Y. 1970. Use of a snake venom toxin to characterize the cholinergic receptor protein. Proc. Nat. Acad. Sci. U.S.A. 67: 1241.

Clementi, F., Whittaker, V. P., and Sheridan, M. N. 1966. The yield of synaptosomes from the cerebral cortex of guinea pigs estimated by a polystyrene bead tagging procedure. Z. Zellforsch. 72: 126.

Coghill, G. E. 1929. Anatomy and the problem of behavior. Macmillan, New York.

Cohen, E. B., and Pappas, G. D. 1969. Dark profiles in the apparently-normal central nervous system. A problem in the electron microscope identification of early anterograde axonal degeneration. J. Comp. Neurol. 136: 375.

Colonnier, M. L. 1966. The structural design of the neocortex, p. 1. In J. C. Eccles (ed.), Pontifica Accademia della Scienze, Rome. Brain and conscious experience. Springer-Verlag, New York.

Corner, M. A., and Crain, S. M. 1969. The development of spontaneous bioelectric activities and strychnine sensitivity during maturation in culture of embryonic chick and rodent central nervous tissues. Arch. Int. Pharmacodyn. Ther. 182: 404.

Corner, M. A., and Crain, S. M. 1972. Patterns of spontaneous bioelectric activity during the maturation in culture of fetal rodent medulla and spinal cord tissues. J. Neurobiol. 3:25.

Coupland, R. E. 1968. Determining sizes and distribution of sizes of spherical bodies such as chromaffin granules in tissue sections. Nature (London) 217: 384.

Cragg, B. G. 1967. The density of synapses and neurones in the motor and visual areas. J. Anat. (London) 101: 639.

Cragg, B. G. 1969. The effects of vision and dark-rearing on the size and density of synapses in the lateral geniculate nucleus measured by electron microscope. Brain Res. 13: 53.

Cragg, B. G. 1970. Synapses and membranous bodies in experimental hypothyroidism. Brain Res. 18: 297.

Cragg, B. G. 1971. The fate of axon terminals in visual cortex during transsynaptic atrophy of the lateral geniculate nucleus. Brain Res. 34: 53.

Crain, S. M. 1964. Development of bioelectric activity during growth of neonatal mouse cerebral cortex in tissue culture, p. 12. In P. Kellaway and I. Petersen (eds.), World Federation of Neurology.

Neurological and electro-encephalographic correlative studies. Grune and Stratton, New York.

Crain, S. M. 1966. Development of "organotype" bioelectric activities in central nervous tissues during maturation in culture. Int. Rev. Neurobiol. 9:1.

Crain, S. M. 1969. Electrical activity of brain tissue developing in culture, p. 506. *In* H. H. Jasper, A. A. Ward, and A. Pope (eds.), Basic mechanisms of the epilepsies. Little, Brown, and Company, Boston.

Crain, S. M. 1970a. Tissue culture studies of developing brain function, p. 165. *In* W. A. Himwich (ed.), Developmental neurobiology. Charles C Thomas, Springfield, Ill.

Crain, S. M. 1970b. Long-term bioelectric studies of spinal cord cultures in closed chamber with sealed-in manipulatable microelectrodes. J. Cell Biol. 47, 2, pt. 2: 43a.

Crain, S. M. 1970c. Bioelectric interactions between cultured fetal rodent spinal cord and skeletal muscles after innervation in vitro. J. Exp. Zool. 173: 353.

Crain, S. M. 1972. Tissue culture models of epileptiform activity, p. 291. *In* D. P. Purpura, J. K. Penry, T. Tower, D. M. Woodbury, and R. Walter (eds.), Experimental models of epilepsy. Raven Press, New York.

Crain, S. M. 1973a. Tissue culture models of developing brain functions. *In* G. Gottlieb (ed.), Developmental studies of behavior and the nervous system, Vol. 2: Aspects of neurogenesis. Academic Press, New York, in press.

Crain, S. M. 1973b. Microelectrode recording in brain tissue cultures. *In* R. F. Thompson and M. M. Patterson (eds.), Methods in physiological psychology, Vol. 1: Bioelectric recording techniques: Cellular processes and brain potentials. Academic Press, New York, in press.

Crain, S. M., and Baer, S. C. 1969. New tissue culture chamber for long-term studies with sealed-in manipulatable microelectrodes. J. Cell Biol. 43, 2, pt. 2: 27a.

Crain, S. M., and Bornstein, M. B. 1964. Bioelectric activity of neonatal mouse cerebral cortex during growth and differentation in tissue culture. Exp. Neurol. 10: 245.

Crain, S. M., and Bornstein, M. B. 1972. Organotypic bioelectric activity in cultured reaggregates of dissociated rodent brain cells. Science 176: 182.

Crain, S. M., Bornstein, M. B., and Peterson, E. R. 1968a. Maturation of cultured embroyonic CNS tissues during chronic exposure to agents which prevent bioelectric activity. Brain Res. 8: 363.

Crain, S. M., Peterson, E. R., and Bornstein, M. B. 1968*b*. Formation of functional interneuronal connections between explants of various mammalian central nervous tissues during development in vitro, p. 13. *In* G. E. W. Wolstenholme and M. O'Connor (eds.), Symposium on growth of the nervous system. A CIBA Foundation symposium.

Crain, S. M., Alfei, L., and Peterson, E. R. 1970. Neuromuscular transmission in cultures of adult human and rodent skeletal muscle after innervation in vitro by fetal rodent spinal cord. J. Neurobiol. 1: 471.

Crain, S. M. and Peterson, E. R. 1967. Onset and development of functional interneuronal connections in explants of rat spinal cord-ganglia during maturation in culture. Brain Res. 6: 750.

Crain, M. S., and Peterson, E. R. 1971. Development of paired explants of fetal spinal cord and adult skeletal muscle during chronic exposure to curare and hemicholinium. In Vitro 6, 5: 373.

Crome, L., and Stern, J. 1967. The pathology of mental retardation. Churchill, London.

Daniels, M. P. 1968. Colchicine inhibition of nerve process elongation in vitro. J. Cell Biol. 39, 2, pt. 2: 21a.

Diamond, J., and Yasargil, G. M. 1969. Synaptic function in the fish spinal cord: Dendritic integration. International symposium on mechanisms of synaptic transmission. Progr. Brain Res. 31: 201.

Eayrs, T. J. 1955. The cerebral cortex of normal and hypothyroid rats. Acta Anat. 25: 160.

Eayrs, T. J. 1966. Thyroid and central nervous development. Sci. Basis Med. Ann. Rev. 317.

Eayrs, T. J., and Taylor, S. H. 1951. The effect of thyroid deficiency induced methyl thiouracil on the maturation of the central nervous system. J. Anat. (London) 85: 350.

Eichenwald, H. F., and Fry, P. C. 1969. Nutrition and learning. Science 163: 644.

Eigsti, O. J., and Dustin, P., Jr. 1955. Colchicine. Iowa State College, Ames.

Feit, H., and Barondes, S. H. 1970. Colchicine-binding activity in particulate fractions of mouse brain. J. Neurochem. 17: 1355.

Feit, H., Dutton, G. R., Barondes, S. H., and Shelanski, M. L. 1971. Microtubule protein: Identification in and transport to nerve endings. J. Cell Biol. 51: 138.

Fifkova, E., and Hassler, R. 1969. Quantitative morphological changes in visual centers in rats after unilateral deprivation. J. Comp. Neurol. 135: 167.

Fuller, J. L., Easler, C. A., and Banks, F. M. 1950. Formation of conditioned avoidance responses in young puppies. Amer. J. Physiol. 160: 462.

Gage, P. W., and Armstrong, C. M. 1968. Miniature end-plate currents in voltage-clamped muscle fibre. Nature (London) 218: 363.

Goldstein, M. N. 1968. Neuroblastoma cells in tissue culture. J. Pediat. Surg. 3: 166.

Grafstein, B. T. 1971. Transneuronal transfer of radioactivity in the central nervous system. Science 172: 177.

Grofova, I., and Rinvik, E. 1970. An experimental electron miscroscopic study on the striatonigral projection in the cat. Exp. Brain Res. 11: 249.

Gruner, J. E. 1970. The maturation of human cerebral cortex in electron microscopy study of post-mortem punctures in premature infants. Biol. Neonate 16: 243.

Guth, L., and Windle, W. F. 1970. The enigma of central nervous regeneration. Summarized transactions of a conference on applications of new technology to the enigma of central nervous regeneration, held in Palm Beach, Florida, February 4–6, 1970, under the auspices of the National Paraplegia Foundation. Exp. Neurol. 28, Suppl. 5: 1.

Gyllensten, L., Malmfors, T., and Norrlin, M. L. 1965. Effect of visual deprivation on the optic centers of growing and adult mice. J. Comp. Neurol. 124: 149.

Ibata, Y., Desiraju, T., and Pappas, G. D. 1971. Light and electron microscopic study of the projection of the medical septal nucleus to the hippocampus of the cat. Exp. Neurol. 33: 103.

Inoue, S., and Sato, H. 1967. Cell motility by labile association of molecules. The nature of mitotic spindle fibers and their role in chromosome movement. J. Gen. Physiol. 50 (Suppl.): 259.

Jones, E. G., and Powell, T. P. S. 1970. An electron microscopic study of the laminar pattern and mode of termination of afferent fibre pathways in the somatic sensory cortex of the cat. Philos. Trans. Roy. Soc. London (Biol. Sci.) 257: 45.

Llinás, R., and Hillman, D. E. 1969. Physiological and morphological organization of the cerebellar circuits in various vertebrates, p. 43. In R. Llinás (ed.), Neurobiology of cerebellar evolution and development. Proceedings of the First International Symposium. American Medical Association, Chicago.

Macklin, M., and Burnett, A. L. 1966. Control of differentiation by calcium and sodium ions in Hydra pseudoligactis. Exp. Cell Res. 44: 665.

Malamud, N. 1964. Neuropathology, p. 429. In H. A. Stevens and R.

Heber (eds.), Mental retardation; A review of research. University of Chicago Press, Chicago.

Marantz, R., and Shelanski, M. L. 1970. Structure of microtubular crystals induced by vinblastine in vitro. J. Cell Biol. 44: 234.

Marin-Padilla, M. 1968. Cortical axo-spinodendritic synapses in man: A Golgi study. Brain Res. 8: 196.

Marotte, L. R., and Mark, R. F. 1970. The mechanism of selective reinnervation of fish eye muscle. II. Evidence from electronmicroscopy of nerve endings. Brain Res. 19: 53.

Miledi, R., Molinoff, P., and Potter, L. T. 1971. Isolation of the cholinergic receptor protein of "Torpedo" electric tissue. Nature (London) 229: 554.

Model, P. G., Bornstein, M. B., Crain, S. M., and Pappas, G. D. 1971. An electron microscopic study of the development of synapses in cultured fetal mouse cerebrum continuously exposed to xylocaine. J. Cell Biol. 49: 326.

Molliver, M. E. 1967. An ontogenetic study of evoked somesthetic cortical responses in the sheep. Developmental neurology. Progr. Brain Res. 26: 78.

Molliver, M. E., and Van der Loos, H. 1970. The ontogenesis of cortical circuitry: The spatial distribution of synapses in somesthetic cortex of new born dogs. Ergeb. Anat. Entwicklungsgesch. 42: 5.

Mountcastle, V. B. 1957. Modality and topographic properties of single neurons of cat's somatic sensory cortex. J. Neurophysiol. 20: 408.

Nelson, P., Ruffner, W., and Nirenberg, M. 1969. Neuronal tumor cells with excitable membranes grown in vitro. Proc. Nat. Acad. Sci. U.S.A. 64: 1004.

Nelson, P. G., Peacock, J. H., Amano, T., and Minna, J. 1971. Electrogenesis in mouse neuroblastoma cells in vitro. J. Cell Physiol. 77: 337.

Noback, C. R., and Purpura, D. P. 1961. Postnatal ontogenesis of neurons in cat neocortex. J. Comp. Neurol. 117: 291.

Olmsted, J. B., Carlson, K., Klebe, R., Ruddle, F., and Rosenbaum, J. 1970. Isolation of microtubule protein from cultured mouse neuroblastoma cells. Proc. Nat. Acad. Sci. U.S.A. 65: 129.

Pappas, G. D. 1966. Electron microscopy of neuronal junctions involved in transmission in the central nervous system, p. 49. In International Research Conference, 4th Lankenau Hospital, Philadelphia. 1964. Nerve as a tissue. Harper & Row, New York.

Pappas, G. D., Cohen, E. B., and Purpura, D. P. 1966. Fine structure of synaptic and nonsynaptic neuronal relations in the thalamus of the cat, p. 46. *In* D. P. Purpura and M. D. Yahr, (eds.), The thalamus. Columbia University Press, New York.

Pappas, G. D., Peterson, E. R., Masurovsky, E. B., and Crain, S. M. 1971. Electron microscopy of the in vitro development of mammalian motor end plates. Ann. N. Y. Acad. Sci. 183: 33.

Payton, B. W., Bennett, M. V. L., and Pappas, G. D. 1969. Permeability and structure of junctional membranes at an electrotonic synapse. Science 166: 1641.

Peterson, E. R., and Crain, S. M. 1970. Innervation in culture of fetal rodent skeletal muscle by organotypic explants of spinal cord from different animals. Z. Zellforsch. 106: 1.

Peterson, E. R., and Crain, S. M. 1972. Regeneration and innervation in cultures of adult mammalian skeletal muscle coupled with fetal rodent spinal cord. Exp. Neurol. 36: 136.

Prechtl, H. F. R. 1958. The directed head turning response to allied movements of the human baby. Behaviour 13: 212.

Purpura, D. P. 1961. Morphophysiological basis of elementary evoked response patterns in the neocortex of the newborn cat. Pavlovian Conference on high nervous activity. Ann. N. Y. Acad. Sci. 92, Art. 3: 840.

Purpura, D. P. 1968. Stability and seizure susceptibility of immature brain, p. 481. *In* Symposium on basic mechanisms of the epilepsies, Colorado Springs. Little, Brown and Company, Boston.

Purpura, D. P. 1972. Intracellular studies of synaptic organizations in the mammalian brain, p. 257. *In* G. D. Pappas and D. P. Purpura (eds.), Structure and function of synapses. Raven Press, New York.

Purpura, D. P., and Housepian, E. M. 1961*a*. Morphological and physiological properties of chronically isolated immature neocortex. Exp. Neurol. 4: 337.

Purpura, D. P., and Housepian, E. M. 1961*b*. Physiological consequences of axon-collateral proliferation in isolated immature neocortex. Fed. Proc. 20: 333.

Purpura, D. P., Prelevic, S., and Santini, M. 1969. Postsynaptic potentials and spike variations in the feline hippocampus during postnatal ontogenesis. Exp. Neurol. 22: 408.

Purpura, D. P., and Shade, J. P. (eds.), 1964. Growth and maturation of the brain. *In* Progr. Brain Res. 4:1 Elsevier Publishing Co., Amsterdam, New York.

Purpura, D. P., Shofer, R. J., and Scarff, T. 1965. Properties of synaptic activities and spike potentials of neurons in immature neocortex. J. Neurophysiol. 28: 925.

Puszkin, E., Puszkin, S., and Aledort, L. M. 1971. Colchicine-binding protein from human patelets and its effect on muscle myosin and platelet myosin-like thrombosthenin-M. J. Biol. Chem. 246: 271.

Ramon-Moliner, E. 1970. The Gogli-cox technique, p. 32. *In* W. N. H. Nauta and S. O. E. Ebbesson (eds.), Contemporary research methods in neuroanatomy. Springer-Verlag, New York.

Ramón y Cajal, S. 1928. Degeneration and regeneration of the nervous system, Vol. I. Translated and edited by Raoul M. May. Oxford University Press, London.

Redburn, D. A., and Dahl, D. R. 1971. Changes in amount of colchicine-binding protein (tubulin) in rabbit brain during development. J. Neurochem. 18: 1689.

Riesen, A. H. 1966. Sensory deprivation. Progr. Physiol. Psychol. 1: 117.

Rosenbaum, J. L., and Carlson, K. 1969. Cilia regeneration in tetrahymena and its inhibition by colchicine. J. Cell Biol. 40: 415.

Schubert, D., and Jacob, F. 1970. 5-Bromodeoxyuridine-induced differentiation of a neuroblastoma. Proc. Nat. Acad. Sci. U.S.A. 67: 247.

Schwartz, I. R., Pappas, G. D., and Purpura, D. P. 1968. Fine structure of neurons and synapses in the feline hippocampus during postnatal ontogenesis. Exp. Neurol. 22: 394.

Seeds, N. W., Gilman, A. G., Amano, T., and Nirenberg, M. W. 1970. Regulation of axon formation by clonal lines of a neural tumor. Proc. Nat. Acad. Sci. U.S.A. 66: 160.

Shelanski, M. L., and Taylor, E. W. 1967. Isolation of a protein subunit from microtubules. J. Cell Biol. 34: 549.

Shelanski, M. L., and Taylor, E. W. 1968. Properties of the protein subunit of central-pair and outer-doublet microtubules of sea urchin flagella. J. Cell Biol. 38: 304.

Shofer, R. J., Pappas, G. D., and Purpura, D. P. 1963. Radiation-induced changes in morphological and physiological properties of immature cerebellar cortex, p. 476. *In* T. J. Haley and R. S. Snider (eds.), International symposium on the response of the nervous system to ionizing radiation, 2nd, Los Angeles, 1963. Little, Brown and Company, Boston.

Sidman, R. L., Dickie, M. M., and Appel, S. H. 1964. Mutant mice (quaking and jumpy) with deficient myelination in the central nervous system. Science 144: 309.

Sidman, R. L., Green, M. C., and Appel, S. H. 1965. Catalog of the neurological mutants of the mouse. Harvard University Press, Cambridge, Mass.

Smith, W. T. 1970. The pathology of the organic dementias. Mod. Trends Neurol. 5: 96.

Stewart, R. M. 1935. Discussion on mental defects from the neurological and psychiatric standpoints. Proc. Roy. Soc. Med. 28: 786.

Taylor, E. W. 1965. The mechanism of colchicine inhibition of mitosis. I. Kinetics of inhibition and the binding of $H^3$-colchicine. J. Cell Biol. 25, 1, pt. 2: 145.

Thesleff, S. 1960. Supersensitivity of skeletal muscle produced by botulinum toxin. J. Physiol. 151: 598.

Valverde, F. 1970. The Golgi method: A tool for comparative structural analyses, p. 12. In W. J. H. Nauta and S. O. E. Ebbesson (eds.), Contemporary research methods in neuroanatomy. Springer-Verlag , New York.

Valverde, F., and Ruiz-Marcos, A. 1969. Dendritic spines in the visual cortex of the mouse: Introduction to a mathematical model. Exp. Brain Res. 8: 269.

Voeller, K., Pappas, G. D., and Purpura, D. P. 1963. Electron microscope study of development of cat superficial neocortex. Exp. Neurol. 7: 107.

Weisenberg, R. C., Borisy, G. G., and Taylor, E. W. 1968. The Colchicine-binding protein of mammalian brain and its relation to microtubules. Biochemistry (Washington) 7: 4466.

Westrum, L. E., White, L. E., Jr., and Ward, A. A., Jr. 1964. Morphology of the experimental epileptic focus. J. Neurosurg. 21: 1033.

Wilson, L. 1970. Properties of colchicine binding protein from chick embryo brain. Interactions with vinca alkaloids and podophyllotoxin. Biochemistry 9: 4999.

Wilson, L., Bryan, L., Ruby, A., and Maxia, D. 1970. Precipitation of proteins by vinblastine and calcium ions. Proc. Nat. Acad. Sci. U.S.A. 66: 807.

Wilson, L., and Friedkin, M. 1967. The biochemical events of mitosis. II. The in vivo and in vitro binding of colchicine in grasshopper embryos and its possible reaction to inhibition of mitosis. Biochemistry (Washington) 6: 3126.

Wisniewski, H., and Terry, R. D. 1967. Experimental colchicine encephalopathy. I. Induction of neurofibrillary degeneration. Lab. Invest. 17: 577.

Wolf, M. K. 1964. Differentiation of neuronal types and synapses in myelinating cultures of mouse cerebellum. J. Cell Biol. 22: 259.

Wolf, M. K. 1970. Anatomy of cultured mouse cerebellum. II. Organotypic migration of granule cells demonstrated by silver impregnation of normal and mutant cultures. J. Comp. Neurol. 140: 281.

Wolf, M. K., and Dubois-Dalcq, M. 1970. Anatomy of cultured mouse cerebellum. I. Golgi and electron microscopic demonstrations of granule cells, their afferent and efferent synapses. J. Comp. Neurol. 140: 261.

Wolf, M. K., and Holden, A. B. 1969. Tissue culture analysis of the inherited defect of central nervous system myelination in jimpy mice. J. Neuropathol. Exp. Neurol. 28: 195.

Yakovlev, P. I. 1959. Anatomy of the human brain and the problem of mental retardation, p. 1. *In* P. W. Bowman and A. Mautner (eds.), International Medical Conference on mental retardation, 1st Portland, Me., Mental retardation. Grune and Stratton, New York.

Zipser, B., Crain, S. M., and Bornstein, M. B. 1973. Intracellular recordings of complex synaptically mediated discharges in explants of fetal hippocampal cortex during maturation in culture. Fed. Proc., in press.

# Index